About the Aut

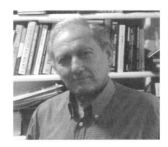

Dr Barry Durrant-Peatfield qualified at Guy's Hospital in 1960 and worked for two years in the Croydon Hospitals before entering general practice. Increasing disenchantment with the NHS decided him to enter private practice where he at once felt drawn to the diagnosis and treatment of thyroid problems. Much impressed by the work of Dr Broda Barnes in the USA, he visited the Barnes Foundation and returned to the UK determined to improve the lot of patients with thyroid illness.

His emphasis on the use of clinical diagnosis, both of thyroid and adrenal problems, and an holistic approach using non-synthetic treatment, enjoyed a great deal of success but brought him into conflict with establishment medicine. And, he finally decided to retire from active medical practice to study nutrition, write and lecture. He wrote the first edition of this book *The Great Thyroid Scandal and How to Survive it* in 2002 for the general reader, to give people a deeper understanding of both thyroid and adrenal illness and enable them to play a knowledgeable role in the management of their treatment. A revised reprint was published in 2003, updating the original. This second, fully revised and updated edition reflects his clinical experience as a nutritional therapist.

Dr Durrant-Peatfield now lectures and holds nutritional clinics specialising in metabolic health.

In loving memory of dear Isabella

Your Thyroid
and
How to Keep it Healthy

Second Edition of
The Great Thyroid Scandal
and How to Survive it

Dr Barry Durrant-Peatfield MB BS LRCP MRCS

Hammersmith Press Ltd
London, UK

First published in Great Britain in 2002, by Barons Down Publishing Ltd, as
The Great Thyroid Scandal and How to Survive it
Revised reprint 2003

Second edition first published in **2006** by Hammersmith Press Limited
14 Greville Street, London, EC1N 8SB
Reprinted 2006, 2007 (twice), 2008 (twice), 2009, 2010 (three times), 2011

www.hammersmithpress.co.uk

Whilst the advice and information in this book are believed to be true and accurate at
the date of going to press, neither the author nor the publisher can accept any
legal responsibility or liability for any errors or omissions that may be made. In
particular (but without limiting the generality of the preceding disclaimer) every
effort has been made to check drug and supplement dosages; however, it is still
possible that errors may have been missed. Furthermore, dosage schedules are
constantly being revised and new side effects recognized. For these reasons
readers are strongly urged to consult printed instructions before taking any drugs or
supplements recommended in this book.

British Library Cataloguing in Publication Data: A CIP record of this book is available
from the British Library.

ISBN 978-1-905140-10-7

Designed by Julie Bennett, Bespoke Publishing
Production by Helen Whitehorn, Pathmedia
Printed and bound by TJ International Ltd of Padstow, Cornwall, UK
Cover image: 'Dame en robe rouge' (Lady in red dress), 1898. By Joszef Rippl-Ronai.
Tapestry, woven by the artist's wife, Lazarine Boudrion. Budapest, Museum of Fine Arts.
Photo: akg-images / Erich Lessing

Contents

Contents

Acknowledgements

Isaac Newton once said that whatever had been his achievements they were because he had stood on the shoulders of giants. This book is founded on the work and vision of men like Dr Murray, Dr Eugene Hertoghe, his grandson Dr Jacques Hertoghe who taught me so much, the pioneer work of Dr Broda Barnes and the extraordinary erudition of Dr John Lowe.

I want to thank those whose commitment to so many seeking help was, and is, always an inspiration, most especially to Lyn Mynott of Thyroid UK.

A debt of gratitude can never be repaid to my staff at my clinic, who worked with such love and care to help our patients through their illness. Especial thanks to Lynn, whose tireless work and devotion knew no bounds. Finally, to Johanne for her patient and painstaking preparation of the manuscript.

Author's Note

I have written this book for the everyday, non-technical reader; yet many of you may well have done a fair amount of personal research into your illness so that much of what you read will be familiar. What seemed to me to be really important is that while being easy to read, you would really like to know some of the more technical aspects of thyroid disease and how they relate to other diseases. There are therefore one or two in-depth explanations which I think will not just be understood, but I hope even enjoyed; and provide you with knowledge you can put to use both in managing your treatment yourself, and enabling you to work in equal partnership with doctors or healthcare practitioners in making decisions about your illness. I have written in the manner I always use in my clinics; that is, that the patient is just as bright as I am, and perfectly able to work things out *given the knowledge*. To give you this knowledge, without clouding it with references within the text or blinding you with science, is I hope what I have been able to do.

The advice offered in this book, although based on my experience with many thousands of patients, is to provide information and my personal opinion. It is not intended to be a substitute for the advice and counsel of your personal physician.

Chapter One

Introduction

In 1877 the great physician William Ord wrote a paper. He had noticed – when he did his post mortems on patients whom he had failed to cure – something wrong with their thyroid gland. His patients had slowly died from a condition which, beginning with general fatigue, weight gain and intractable coldness, had progressed to hair loss, bloating, extreme constipation, depression, loss of thinking powers and muscle and joint stiffness. It seemed that every system in their body slowed down and stopped; some patients slipped into coma, some into madness. But they all died, sometimes taking years and years in the process. He found that the thyroid (which as most people know sits in the neck on either side of the Adam's apple) was atrophied, shrunken, scarred and fibrous. Obviously it wasn't working. Ord coined the term myxoedema as a name for the illness he was describing. The 'oedema' (swelling) was because the skin looked bloated and puffy; the 'myx' because although the puffiness looked like water it was actually water bound in a protein material, called mucin, which could not be drained off or treated.

Various treatments were tried. Some patients, with enlargement of the neck, got better if they were given elemental iodine. Some didn't. Eventually, Murray, in 1892, hit upon a solution: since the thyroid was atrophying or shrinking by degrees, why not grind up healthy thyroid glands from animals; all mammals have thyroid glands. By 1898 he was giving this ground-up thyroid by mouth. It may sound horrible and disgusting – but two ladies, apparently terminally ill with all the symptoms we mentioned above, started getting better. Soon it was clear they were cured – until the extract was stopped. He had discovered the cure for hypothyroidism. As the years passed, researchers worked out how to dry, or desiccate, the animal thyroid, so it could be put into tablet form. This desiccated thyroid is widely used today, especially in the USA; and in the UK, following its complete disuse by 1985, it is now returning.

We must turn back to 1914 when, in a masterly exposition, the great Belgian physician Eugene Hertoghe, described, as only the great physicians of the past can, the illness and how to diagnose and to treat it. It has been my great privilege to know and be taught by his grandson Jacques; and his children Thierry and Theresa Hertoghe carry on the work. He described a number of patients, men and women, in whom a bewildering variety of symptoms presented themselves; sometimes the patients were mildly ill and sometimes very ill. For a moment we can listen to his words.

"When you encounter the association of one or more of the following symptoms: trophic changes [basically loss of normal health] in hair, eyebrows, eyelashes, teeth or gums; an habitual chilliness, biliary disturbances with cholelithiasis [gallstones], dyspnoea [breathlessness] with asthma attacks, menorrhagia [heavy periods], recurring abortion [miscarriage], haemophilia [bleeding and bruising tendency], melancholic depression, weariness of life, migraine, vertigo, sudden loss of consciousness, noises in the ear, somnolence, rheumatoid changes in the muscles or ligaments, loss of appetite, obstinate constipation – think of possible deficiency of thyroid secretion."

We shall add other symptoms as we progress.

We owe an enormous debt to the life's work of the great American physician Dr Broda Barnes. He began his work in the early 1930s when he studied the thyroid for his doctorate. He became a practising physician and devoted his life to bringing to the attention of doctors the true nature of hypothyroidism, and treating thousands of grateful patients. He was continually on the move, lecturing and exhibiting, and wrote many papers for medical journals. He carried on into the 1980s and founded the Barnes Foundation (Trumbull, Connecticut) to continue his work. He died in 1989 leaving behind an immense body of work and the Foundation, which is actively in existence today. It was at the Foundation that my own beliefs and anxieties about hypothyroidism found their full focus.

Towards the end of his life, he and another brilliant physician, Dr William McCormack Jeffries, met and brought their own specialised fields together. Jeffries' seminal work, *The Safe Uses of Cortisone*, showed the world that cortisone, far from being the ogre which patients and doctors have come to regard it, was entirely essential in the treatment of a number of illnesses. It played a vital role, as we shall see, in the successful treatment of thyroid disease.

It perhaps goes without saying, that both these great physicians have not had the attention and regard from the medical profession as a whole that they deserve. You would think that their painstaking research, carefully conducted trials and many published papers could not be ignored but very largely they have been. Convention is a hard and implacable enemy. Nevertheless, as you will see in this book, my experience has shown they *were* right. To what extent this occurs in other scientific circles is difficult to say; but medicine is notorious for its vilification of new thought and discoveries. One must recall, with a wry smile, poor William Harvey, in the reign of Queen Elizabeth I, who concluded that the heart pumped blood around the body. In those days they didn't mess about; he had a contract put out on him and had to leave the country for 10 years. When Ignaz Semmelweiss had the appalling effrontery to suggest that the high death rate (in early Victorian times) of recently delivered mothers from puerperal fever would be lessened if doctors *washed their hands* after dissecting their failures, before going to the delivery room, the profession scorned him as an interfering charlatan. There are, sadly, many others who have similarly suffered. And, things haven't changed much have they? Think about MRSA.

However, in this day and age the work must go on. We owe a great deal to Dr John Lowe in the USA, whose monumental and deeply researched *The Metabolic Treatment of Fibromyalgia* should be set reading for all endocrinologists everywhere. Especially, be it said, in the United Kingdom. I have myself been treating patients for hypothyroidism and the low adrenal reserve syndrome for some 25 years and have learnt much. Most especially, I have learned how to make people better and empowered them to help themselves and others.

Since the advent of the internet the situation has undergone dramatic change. Mary Shomon in the USA must be known through her website to millions all over the world. So too must Dr Joseph Mercola – from Armour Pharmaceuticals – also a household name in America. There are others; very well known are the Doctors Teitelbaum and Goldstein who too have their websites. This has enabled people to teach themselves about their illness.

The problem of course is that it is one thing knowing what is actually wrong, but it is quite another getting your doctor or endocrinologist to treat you. The literature for popular reading, which is extensive and well informed, is sadly dismissed out of hand by so many healthcare practitioners. The number of research articles is colossal and there can be no excuse on the part of any physician for not recognising and treating any patient with thyroid illness who seeks their help. But, disgracefully, many of these remain unread and not acted upon. A second problem is that many papers are designed to express a point of view. If as a researcher or practising physician you are convinced that thyroid dysfunction is actually not very common and anyway admirably treated, it is not actually very difficult to use statistics to prove your point. "There are lies, more lies and damned statistics", as Mark Twain wrote. However well researched a paper on the use, say, of natural thyroid, the same problem may arise; and since these papers are in contravention of established belief, they may be regarded as frank heresy. In any event, a confusing picture emerges and a doctor is obliged to follow conventional thinking, or reap the consequences. This approach means that many thousands of patients yearly are either undiagnosed altogether or inadequately treated. These latter may well improve somewhat, for some time, but *they are never as well as they should be*. And when you consider the figure for people developing low thyroid function may well be 30% and not 2% or 5% as I have seen quoted by many supposed experts in the field, you can have an idea of the immensity of the problem: the years of ill-health suffered unnecessarily by so many; and the fact that low thyroid function means premature ageing and death from heart disease, stroke, diabetes, cancer and other illnesses of advancing age.

Time, I think, to explore why the thyroid goes wrong. To begin we can find out how it is made and what it does.

Chapter Two

How It Works

The thyroid gland is one of a family of glands collectively called the endocrine system. Endocrines secrete within themselves complex molecules called hormones (from the Greek "hormon", meaning to stir up, which is just what they do). These hormones pass into the bloodstream, where they act as chemical messengers, targeting other glands or organs or tissues, and telling them what to do. Vital functions of the body are controlled in this way, the endocrine glands responding to the needs of the moment. (To avoid confusion, the other group of glands, called exocrine glands, pass their secretions straight to the site of action as for example, the salivary glands.)

Now have a glance at Figure 1, which shows where these very special glands are situated. Working from the top downwards, the first is the pea-sized pineal gland. This is deep within our brains covered by the cerebral cortex. The interesting thing is that in primitive animals, like certain reptiles, it's actually so near the top of the skull that it can respond to light. Eastern mystics, even now, refer to it as the third eye. In us humans, it can still respond to light but by way of the optic nerves which pass very close to it.

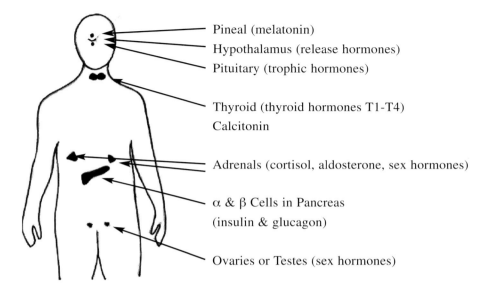

Pineal (melatonin)
Hypothalamus (release hormones)
Pituitary (trophic hormones)

Thyroid (thyroid hormones T1-T4)
Calcitonin

Adrenals (cortisol, aldosterone, sex hormones)

α & β Cells in Pancreas
(insulin & glucagon)

Ovaries or Testes (sex hormones)

Figure 1. The Endocrine System

The pineal gland produces mostly the hormone melatonin and has some influence over the hypothalamus (which comes next). It is the gland that controls our bodily (or circadian) rhythms, both short and long term. For example, as the day wears on, and the shadows fall, it produces melatonin, which shuts down our biological mechanisms so that we can drift off to sleep. There are other rhythms: those controlling, for example, seasonal activity. In some animals, hibernation; in humans, the young man's fancy in the spring. The longest rhythm of all is the ageing process and the timing of when to call a halt to all our trials and tribulation. There is more about the hormone melatonin itself in Chapter Seven.

Below the pineal in the floor of the brain, is the hypothalamus. This is part brain and part endocrine gland. It is the interface between our endocrine system and what is going on in the outside world, as passed to it from the input of our senses via the brain. Hence we can control to a degree, albeit largely unconsciously, our endocrine system.

To exert this control over the endocrine system as a whole, the hypothalamus raps out its instructions to the pituitary gland attached by a stalk just below it. These instructions come as 'release' hormones, which the pituitary must obey; and it responds by producing hormones of its own, the 'trophic' hormones, which are passed through the bloodstream to other endocrine glands, or tissues.

The endocrine system can be likened to an orchestra; with the pituitary as the conductor and the hypothalamus as the composer of the wonderful symphony of life. In the stalls sits the director, the pineal, hissing out instructions and criticism… and finally, perhaps ordering the fall of the curtain.

Anterior   **Posterior**

ACTH (adrenocorticotrophic hormone)
GH   (growth hormone)   Vasopressin (ADH)
HPL   (human placental lactogen)   (Anti-diuretic hormone)
PL   (prolactin)
LH   (luteinising hormone)   Oxytocin
FSH   (follicle stimulating hormone)
TSH   (thyroid stimulating hormone)
MSH   (melanocyte stimulating hormone)

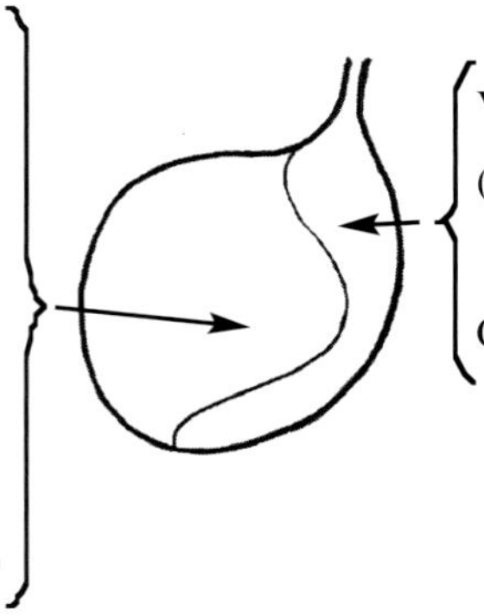

Figure 2. The Pituitary Gland

So let us look now at the conductor, the pituitary gland. If you have a look at Figure 2, you will see that it has a front (anterior) half and a back (posterior) half. The front is really quite busy, and produces many different hormones. Since these don't all concern us at the moment, I am not going to go into any detail about them, but I have listed them for those of you who are interested. However, two of them must catch our attention at once: the thyroid stimulating hormone (TSH), of which a good deal more later, and the adrenocorticotrophic hormone (ACTH), which controls adrenal function. The luteinising hormone (LH) and follicle stimulating hormone (FSH), control the female hormones and the menstrual cycle in the ladies, and the male hormones and spermatozoa formation in the lads.

To show how all this works let us take a look at the thyroid gland. Suppose we find that we are cold and miserable. The hypothalamus responds to this by making the thyrotrophin release hormone (TRH). This is now passed via the bloodstream to the pituitary gland, which then makes the TSH. And this, as we see in Figure 3, gets the thyroid going to produce more thyroid hormone, which increases our metabolic activity and helps us warm up.

Since later on I shall be discussing adrenal function, I can illustrate how this works in the same way. The adrenal glands can produce many different hormones, but the two we are concerned about here are adrenaline (or epinephrine in the US) and noradrenaline (norepinephrine) – the fight or flight hormones – and cortisol, which enable the body to cope with stress; acute stress for the adrenalins, longer-term stress for the cortisones – for example, illness or severe external stress. The hypothalamus is made aware of the stress situation and produces the corticotrophin release hormone (CRH), which stimulates the pituitary to produce ACTH and so the adrenals are instructed to produce extra cortisol.

So we have an elegant negative feedback mechanism to control the target endocrine glands. (A negative feedback is much the same as your central heating at home. As the water in the radiators gets hotter, eventually a sensor shuts off the gas.) The feedback works because the hypothalamus is monitoring the blood levels of the hormones concerned as well as external inputs; in the case of the thyroid hormone

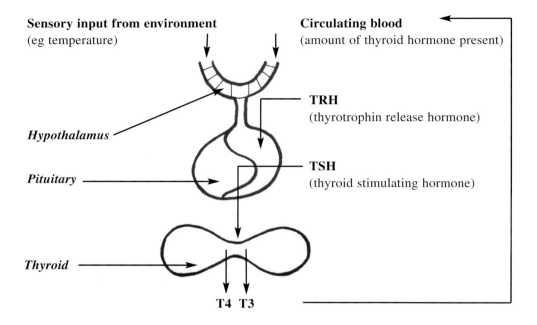

Sensory input from environment
(eg temperature)

Circulating blood
(amount of thyroid hormone present)

TRH
(thyrotrophin release hormone)

Hypothalamus

Pituitary

TSH
(thyroid stimulating hormone)

Thyroid

T4 T3

Figure 3. Trophic Hormone Feedback Loop

when blood levels are optimum the release hormone production is shut down and, via the pituitary, the target gland production is also shut down. The adrenal control is clearly the same.

There are few people who don't know that the thyroid gland is in the neck, developing very early in foetal life. It has two lobes, which meet across the windpipe at about the level of the Adam's apple, and is 3 or 4 inches across. Usually these lobes are not really visible, although they can be felt; but in some thyroid conditions they enlarge, sometimes very much, and are easily seen. They can also become inflamed, when they are painful to the touch. Cysts and growths may from time to time occur and they too may be seen and felt. Abnormally large thyroids may be quite uncomfortable and interfere with swallowing and speech.

The function of the thyroid, in us and all mammals, is to regulate all the processes of energy release within individual cells and in the body as a whole. (The thyroid hormones also act as growth hormones controlling tissue growth and development in early life.) This is what we mean when we talk about metabolism. Metabolism is the rate at which we produce and use energy. The release of energy from life processes in its simplest terms is the combination of oxygen from the air we breathe, with hydrocarbons from our food. These are molecules made up of chains of carbon and hydrogen atoms. One of the simplest is of course sugar and all the carbohydrates we eat are turned into the sugar glucose. By complex processes, fats and proteins can also be turned into glucose when required. All this happens within each individual cell, using complex enzymes operating within a miniature energy generating station called the mitochondrion. Here the magic occurs; the carbon and hydrogen atoms are released to combine with the oxygen, forming carbon dioxide (CO_2) and water (H_2O). This process releases chemical energy, which is what the cell lives on.

Now the thyroid hormone works on this process in two principle ways. First, it assists the enzyme systems that enable these nutrients, and also electrolytes like sodium, potassium and other chemicals, to pass into the cell itself through its protective membrane. (It also works in the reverse manner to allow the waste products to diffuse out.) But its chief importance lies in facilitating the processes of energy production in the mitochondria. So any lack of thyroid hormone reduces overall energy production. (Of course, too much can increase energy production above normal.) These effects are readily seen and complained of by the patient.

So now we need to have a look at this magic chemical, the thyroid hormone. Actually, there are four thyroid hormones produced by the thyroid gland; but most of the work is done by one of them, the one called *tri-iodothyronine (T3)* which I explain below. The process is this. Within the colloid spaces of the thyroid – divided up into 10 or 12 compartments – the thyroid hormones are made. In the presence of the thyroid stimulating hormone (TSH) and the thyroperoxidase (TPO) enzyme, and the element selenium, the ringed amino acid tyrosine has one or two iodine atoms added to it. (This is called iodination.) One, or two, iodine atoms make the new compounds mono-iodotyrosine (MIT) or di-iodotyrosine (DIT). The cunning bit is that now these compounds join up, actually on top of one another (although in the diagrams (Figures 4-8) I have shown them flattened out). Joined up like this, they have become thyronine compounds, and may then have no iodine atoms in their structure, or one, or two, or three, or four, depending on how many iodine atoms were on each tyrosine ring – none, one, or two. About 80% of the thyroid output into the bloodstream is in the T4 version; about 16% as T3 and the remaining 4% made up of T2 and T1.

Shown below in Figure 4 is **thyroxine (T4)**.

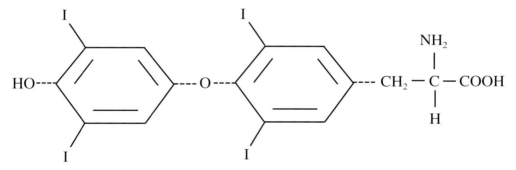

Figure 4. (T4) 3,5,3',5'-tetra-iodothyronine

If we take away one of the iodine atoms, we have **tri-iodothyronine (T3)**.

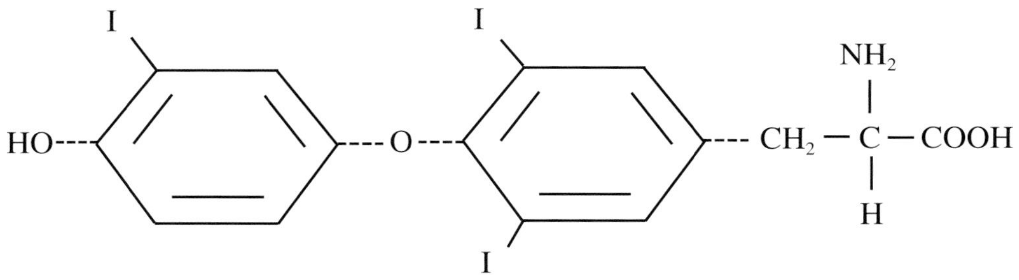

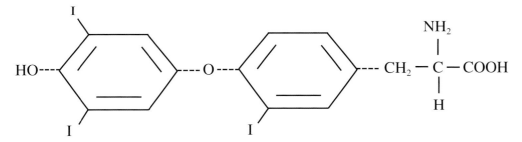

Figure 5. (T3) 3,5,3'-tri-iodothyronine (liothyronine)

If a different iodine is removed, as in Figure 6, we have an isomer of T3, (same number of atoms, but arranged differently) called **reverse T3 (rT3)**.

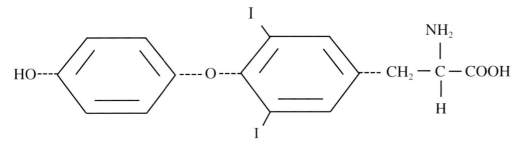

Figure 6. (rT3) 3,3',5'-tri-iodothyronine

With two iodine atoms removed we have **di-iodothyronine (T2)**. (The two iodine atoms may be on the first or second ring, or one on each ring.)

Figure 7. (T2) 3,5-di-iodothyronine

With only one iodine atom, we now have **mono-iodothyronine (T1)**. The iodine atom may appear on the first or second ring.

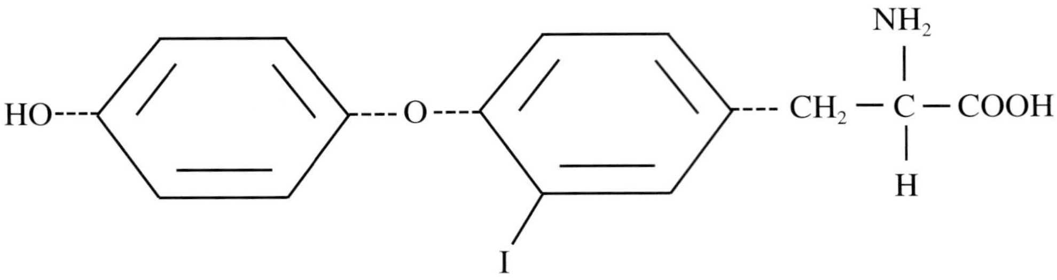

Figure 8. (T1) 3-mono-iodothyronine

What I think is interesting is how very similar the molecules are; unless you knew, you would have to look hard to see the differences, and yet they have totally different effects in the body. It all depends on how many iodine atoms there are, and where they go. So let's have a look at them and see what they do.

First, the thyroxine or T4. Although the thyroid gland makes more of this than the others, it actually has a low biological activity and, as it stands its effect is minimal. The T4 gets attached to a protein transport compound and is whirled around the body in the bloodstream in temporary storage, awaiting as it were, the call of duty. In this form it is only slowly used up and has a 'half-life' of about 8 days. This means that after 8 days there is half the amount left; and 8 further days later, half of that. And so on. So if the body is not continuing to produce the correct amount, there is still some left after 4 to 6 weeks, but not very much.

As I have already said, the thyroid hormone that does all the work is tri-iodothyronine or liothyronine (T3). It works like this. If we suppose that there is a need for increased energy production (say we have gone out into the cold without a coat and we need to heat up) then the thyroid gland will soon produce more T4 and more T3. The T3 is used by the tissues for increased energy production at once; but as it gets used up, the T4 is now called upon and one of three 5'-deiodinase enzymes rapidly removes one of the four iodine molecules from the T4 and converts it into the active T3, which can then get to work increasing energy production (and hence heat) from the tissues – most of the conversion takes place in the liver. But what can also happen is that one of the other 5'-deiodinase enzymes can remove a different iodine atom as in Figure 6, and this forms reverse T3, which I have written about in detail in Chapter Eleven. For now, all we need say is that reverse T3 has no biological activity in the control of metabolism.

So far as clinical medicine goes it is T3 and T4 that mostly concern us. T2, otherwise known for those who wish to be technical, as 3,5-di-iodo-L-thyronine, has received increasing attention from research workers of late. Previously thought to have only a role in passing, as part of the upward pathway from T1 to T3 and T4 or part of a degradation process to recycle iodine, it now seems that T2 actually has a number of important supplementary roles to play.

First of all, it has recently been found that T2 has a stimulatory effect on the activity of the 5'-deiodinase enzyme, encouraging the production of T3. As T3 is produced it exerts an inhibitory effect on the production of TSH by the pituitary; an example of a negative feedback loop. It turns out that this inhibitory effect is much reduced where T2 is concerned, which may have metabolic advantages.

It was shown that T2 alone is effective in increasing liver metabolism and also that of heart, muscle tissue and brown adipose tissue.[1] (This is brown fat, where surplus calories are burnt away rather than being deposited in the fat stores.) It is as good as, or even better than, T3 in liver and lipid (fat) metabolism.[2] I think that it is more than likely that T2 will be shown to have a significantly greater effect than has hitherto been thought. T2 is not given by any doctors in the United Kingdom; but it is of course part of the natural desiccated thyroid supplements we shall be talking about in due course. This is perhaps why they work so much better than T4 or T3 on their own.

New products have become available, very recently, that make use of another property of T2. It turns out that T2 can enhance catabolism (that is the breakdown) of body fat without breaking down muscle tissue as well. It is therefore used in weight loss programmes, where an increased metabolism is required without muscle loss. (These products come from the USA and so far do not have FDA accreditation.)

The production of thyroid hormones, and their transport around the system in the bloodstream, all depend on a proper balance of raw materials, and enzymes controlling their use. Enzymes are complex substances that mediate all sorts of chemical processes; like the hormones themselves, they also require various raw materials to make them and to help them work. For the manufacture of thyroid hormones a healthy, varied and, wherever possible, organic diet is needed. There are things you should eat, and things you shouldn't.

Things you shouldn't eat in large quantities are called goitrogenic foods. The brassicas, cabbage and brussel sprouts for example, contain thiouracil, which inhibits the actual manufacture of thyroid hormone within the gland. Others are, turnips, cassava, pine nuts, mustard, peanuts and millet. However, good English cooking tends to destroy these goitrogens. Soya beans have high levels of phyto-oestrogens, which can reduce the amount of thyroid hormone available from its transport protein. Another common foodstuff to be thought about is, I am sorry to say, tea, since it contains significant levels of fluoride, which has a damaging effect on thyroid manufacture and tissue uptake.

Needed, are proteins, which contain the amino acid phenylalanine that converts to tyrosine (see Chapter Nine). We learnt earlier that there has to be enough of the amino acid tyrosine, the basis of thyroid hormone.

There also has to be enough iodine to join up with the tyrosine. Iodine has been known as necessary for thyroid hormone production since ancient times: Egyptian physicians gave their tired and overweight patients seaweeds and sponges. Although iodine makes the thyroid hormone actually do the work to control metabolism, too much will cause thyroid suppression. Iodine foodstuffs are required in moderation: having said that, the amount of iodine depends on the iodine levels of the soil in which they are grown and our soils, especially inland, are short of iodine. Professor Hume of Dundee a few years ago carried out an interesting and worrying study on a number of expectant mothers.[3] He found 40% of them were short of iodine. This is important, since this deficiency can affect development of the baby's nervous system.

And there has to be enough of the metal selenium to help in the joining up process. It is also the basis of the 5'-deiodinase enzymes, which regulate the manufacture of the active T3 from the T4. Without these, the thyroid cannot make, and we cannot use, thyroid hormones. It is essential as an antioxidant and in the proper working of the immune system. Selenium levels are also low in our foodstuffs on the whole.

But it doesn't end there. The enzymes cannot do their job without a number of other chemical substances. These are called co-factors. For thyroid hormone manufacture and its use, these have to be present as well. There are quite a few of them. First, there are the minerals: magnesium, manganese, zinc, chromium, iron, copper and calcium. We don't need a lot, but they must be there. Secondly, there are the vitamins. Really, they are all needed; but especially we need the B complex vitamins, including vitamin B$_{12}$ and folic acid. We need vitamins A and E; and most especially vitamin C.

We now have a working knowledge of the thyroid gland, its hormones and what they do. We must now find out how it can go wrong and why and what we can do about it.

Chapter Three

When Things Go Wrong – Part 1

The Over-active Thyroid Gland and Its Treatment

The beautifully balanced biochemical mechanism I have described in Chapter Two can maintain us in perfect health all our lives. Sadly, however, it may go out of kilter, sometimes quite abruptly, and sometimes insidiously slowly, causing a slow decline in health and vigour, which will inexorably destroy people's lives. On the one hand the thyroid gland can become over-active, bringing with it a variety of unpleasant, even life-threatening symptoms, or it may become under-active causing a bewildering number of problems, varying from mere loss of energy and vigour to chronic invalidism and sudden death. We will look first at over-activity.

There are two groups of problems which can move the thyroid into an over-active state. Firstly, there may be a control problem. This can originate right at the top of the chain of command. The hypothalamus may produce too much of the thyrotrophin release hormone (TRH), thus causing over-activity in TSH production, and hence over-activity of the thyroid itself. For example, the cells responsible for TRH production may overwork, as in the case of a hormone producing cancer, called an adenoma. Fortunately, not very common. But there may be over-stimulation of these cells from the brain itself. High levels of stress from major life events can be responsible. Young adults, especially women, may be subject to this. Or the TRH producing cells may become insensitive to circulating thyroid hormone and overproduce to compensate.

More commonly, the pituitary itself may start producing more TSH. This can occur as a result of a pituitary adenoma, the growth producing the hormone in an uncontrolled fashion. There may be a genetic problem with these cells, which may escape from the proper controls and start doing their own thing. Or, they can become oversensitive to hypothalamic TRH, with the same result. Whatever the cause, the thyroid becomes over-stimulated and more thyroid hormone is produced than is required.

Most causes of overproduction of thyroid hormone, however, occur in the gland itself. The receptors which respond to TSH may over-respond and react by overproducing thyroid hormones. The body itself makes antibodies to the thyroid tissue, which initially may cause overproduction of thyroid hormone, but in time, this effect may burn itself out and then the receptors become insensitive and thyroid production starts to become affected the other way, resulting eventually in underproduction of thyroid hormone. This problem of antibodies as a cause of illness, applies not just to the thyroid, but other organs and tissues as well. I have explained it in more detail later in the section on Hashimoto's disease.

For reasons that may not be clear, but again are sometimes the result of major traumatic life events, the thyroid-producing cells simply overproduce. The thyroid may become subject to an inflammatory process – thyroiditis – which may run its course to leave the thyroid normal again, or subject perhaps, to an instability between over and under-activity.

The over-active thyroid, **hyperthyroidism**, was first described as far back as 1835, by an Irish physician, Robert Graves; and a German physician, Karl von Basedow, hastened to write a paper about it in 1840. Hence in the UK we call it Graves' disease, and the Europeans, Basedow's disease. The thyroid gland is usually enlarged and clearly visible, a condition most often seen in young women. As a whole, women are more often affected than men, usually in the younger age groups; but it may occur at any age and in either sex. It is known to be the result of autoimmune antibody attack and is for this reason also called autoimmune thyroiditis. In general it is diagnosed without difficulty. The treatment of Graves' disease, however, is often not at all satisfactory. So let's have a closer look.

Symptoms

The patient will appear nervous and anxious as a general rule, and indeed may be thought to be suffering from anxiety only. Most patients will be losing weight in spite of a good appetite, although occasionally they may be anorexic (without appetite). They complain of frequent and loose bowel action. They tend to be breathless and though often hyperactive, tired at the same time. There is a usual complaint of feeling hot much of the time, always turning down the heating, and they become aware of palpitations, either because the heart beats too fast or the pulse has become irregular.

Signs

The doctor will look for the following. Weight loss may well be apparent in a number of patients, but certainly not all. There may be staring eyes, the result of the fat behind the eyes swelling partly with fluid; this is called exophthalmos. One classic sign is lid-lag, where the doctor asks the patients to look at his finger as he rapidly drops it in front of their vision. The upper lid lags behind the eye following the finger. The pulse will be rapid, sometimes irregular, and the hand will be unexpectedly warm to the touch; obvious too, will be a tremor of the hand. The extra blood flow to the thyroid can sometimes be picked up by the doctor through his stethoscope; he can hear a rushing noise, which is called the 'thyroid bruit'. The blood pressure will be revealing too: the upper (systolic) value will be unusually widely separated from the lower (diastolic) value. Another typical finding is pretibial myxoedema, a puffiness apparent over the bone of the lower leg.

Armed with all this information, the diagnosis should be clear. Confirmatory blood tests will show abnormally high T4 and/or T3 levels, and abnormally low TSH, which together with the presence of antibodies (TgAb) will suggest autoimmune thyroiditis. Clearly, the diagnosis in general isn't difficult to make. The rub comes in the treatment.

Treatment

First, you may not have to do very much. Mild degrees of thyroid over-activity can occur on a self-limiting basis, and may sometimes be left to run their own course, with an informed patient monitoring how they are, and seeking equally well-informed advice if things are not going right. The body has a remarkable ability to heal itself, and should be given the chance to do so. The most successful early physicians knew their subject so well that the natural course, and eventual self-healing of the illness, was often quite predictable. So the "Vital Elixir" was given just before the patient showed clear signs of getting better, with of course, miraculous results. This incidentally, is not the same as the placebo effect (often cited as the result of thyroid and adrenal therapy), which occurs for a limited time as a result of strong suggestion by the prescriber or high expectation by the patient. Sometimes a remarkable and dramatic recovery occurs using eye of newt and toe of frog. This bedevils a balanced judgement of cause and effect.

Sorry, I digress.

So the first approach is an alert and informed assessment of progress, intervening only when necessary. Over-intervention is the curse of modern medicine in almost any illness you can imagine; we should take to heart that sometimes a policy of 'masterly inactivity' is much better for the patient and may even spare his life.

The second line of approach is to relieve symptoms until it is clear that the illness is either going to resolve itself in time or will require sterner measures. There are two medical weapons in most common use. First, simple anxiolytics. These are basically tranquillisers, and are acceptable for a limited time where the degree of over-activity causes nervous tremor, worry, panic and palpitations. The old-fashioned, and much derided Valium has a use here – not a large dose, say 5 mg twice or three times a day – can make life bearable. Along with this or possibly instead, 'beta-blockers' may be used. These are a group of compounds which prevent high levels of nervous activity reaching the tissues, and have a general calming effect on anxiety, nervous shaking and rapid pulse, in addition to their other therapeutic effects like reducing blood pressure, slowing down heart action (helping angina) and preventing migraines. The one most widely used is Propranolol, often 10 to 40 mg two or three times a day, according to need. Even with extensive use there are very few either short-term or long-term side effects, although asthma is sometimes a problem. Many doctors have found that a combination of an anxiolytic and a beta-blocker, in really small doses, works better than high doses of either by themselves and may control mild hyperthyroidism for extended periods of time.

When things are getting tougher, the next approach is the use of a chemical block on the production within the thyroid of thyroxine, which prevents the iodine molecules from attaching themselves normally to the thyronine molecule. Two preparations have been in use for years: the commonest is carbimazole (usually in multiples of 5 mg) and the other is propyl-thiouracil (20 mg). They are both widely used as a bulwark against invasive surgical or medical attack, as I will discuss in a moment. There are of course difficulties: they have been found to cause problems with the growth of white blood cells, suddenly and unexpectedly, and the immune system may be so compromised that a major or minor infection may suddenly appear. Sometimes, of course, the patient is simply intolerant of the medication and becomes ill.

A regular daily dose is chosen; rapidly, the amount of thyroid hormone production starts to fall, and the circulation of thyroid hormone starts to decline. The trick, of course, is to ensure the dose is neither too much, nor too little, remembering that thyroid production and thyroid hormone requirement may vary quite a lot. If this isn't borne in mind, the result will be that the patient may be out of balance, either over or under-active. Most physicians fall back on the blood test to adjust doses, but I think it is tiresome to have repeated tests, when the patient – who after all, knows how they feel better than anybody – may often have a much better idea of their requirements than any blood test. I have always taught my patients to check their pulse rate once or twice a day and their resting temperature; and to make an overall assessment as to whether they feel well or not. If too much of the medicine is given, the thyroid activity will be low and the patient will feel tired, cold and sluggish; the pulse may be low, say 60 beats a minute; the resting temperature below 36.6°C or 97.8°F. (Of this resting temperature more anon.) The patient should in my view, with ordinary commonsense, then adjust the dose downwards (or have a day or so off) until things have put themselves right. And, of course vice versa.

This treatment may be used for an extended time – certainly a year or so – so long as the self-monitoring and the advice from an understanding doctor or healthcare practitioner provide for virtual normality. Most commonly, the over-active state will, with ups and downs, tend to correct itself; and the patient may find in time the medication becomes unnecessary. A life event or illness may, however, start it all over again, but the patient by now will recognise the symptoms and be able to deal with them. Another common sequel however, is that having normalised for a while, the thyroid activity may start running below normal. This as we noted before occurs with Hashimoto's disease. The management problem is that this running down may be slow and insidious; the loss of energy and well-being, the weight gain, may go more or less unnoticed, may be put down to age, overwork, worry, or bad eating, before it becomes obvious that all is not well. Informed patients – and that is what this book is about – will alert themselves to this and seek advice. This may or may not be helpful, and patients may have to take matters into their own hands, using available natural thyroid support not requiring a prescription. I will elaborate on this later (see Chapter Nine.)

Popular in some quarters is the 'block and replace' approach to treatment. A dose of carbimazole (Neomercazole) or propyl-thiouracil is chosen to be deliberately in excess of the actual requirements – enough more or less to shut the whole thing down. Then, thyroxine is added to bring it all back to normal. Yes, I know what you're thinking. However, the idea is to shut the thyroid down so thoroughly that it is sufficiently shocked by it all not to relapse when the anti-thyroid treatment is withdrawn. It is claimed that control is smoother, and there is a lower relapse rate. All I can say is that it may work this way sometimes, but it's difficult to be convinced.

What should be the final solution is in my view all too rapidly turned to by doctors and surgeons, who may consider their solution the treatment of choice right from the start. It has the merit of usually having an immediate effect, but may bring in its train other problems, and simply exchange one therapeutic master for another, with no hope of a normal thyroid function without continuous and long-term medication. This final solution is thyroid ablation, which means the thyroid is knocked out finally and forever.

Two approaches are chosen: the first is radioactive iodine. Here I_{131}, the radioactive form, is given to the patient as a drink. The radioactive iodine concentrates in the thyroid tissue and 'nukes it'. The second is surgery, where a proportion of thyroid tissue is removed. The problem with these two solutions lies in their permanence; they cannot be undone, and getting it right, that is 'nuking', or removing the right amount, can only be a matter of guesswork. More often than not, the amount destroyed or removed is not right to begin with; furthermore, it obviously cannot allow for changes in thyroid function which will occur with the passage of time.

With radioactive iodine ablation there is the merit of simplicity. A solution is prepared of the radioactive isotope of iodine (I_{131}), which is swallowed in one draught. The thyroid uses iodine as its main raw material as we saw, and so this radioactive form concentrates in the colloid (hormone forming) tissue in the thyroid gland. (Of course, it goes elsewhere in the body, especially the breast. But you may not be told this.) We all know that radioactivity destroys cells and Chernobyl showed us how terrible its uncontrolled effects are. I_{131} concentrates itself in the cells and its radioactivity destroys them. The severity of cellular damage depends, of course, on how much is initially given. This amount is calculated by body weight and the presumed severity of the over-activity of the thyroid forming cells. You hope it is about right… You have undergone all the blood tests after all. And we know blood tests are wonderful and right… Or do we?

There are three possible scenarios. One is that the calculation was right – it does happen. The amount of thyroid tissue left is just right to produce the right level of hormones in the bloodstream. (Of course the cells may later partly recover, and then it may have to be done all over again or further damage and loss of function may occur and the thyroid as a whole may become under-active.)

The second scenario is that the patient continues to have an over-active thyroid in spite of treatment, and a further dose of radioactive iodine – or doses – may have to be given at once. In this circumstance, getting it right becomes more and more unlikely.

The third scenario is a good deal more common. Overkill becomes evident in a few days, and thyroid hormone in the bloodstream falls pretty quickly. Very soon thyroid replacement (usually thyroxine) becomes necessary. So long as the physician is convinced that this is what has happened – admits it, in spite of blood tests which may or may not confirm the situation – and prescribes thyroxine, the resulting hypothyroidism can be sorted out. However, as we shall see later, diagnosis is most likely to be based on blood levels, and not on what the patient is saying. So the hapless patient, bewildered by this perfect high tech wonder treatment, repeatedly assured how much better they must be, but feeling more or less terrible, exchanges one sort of pill for another, this time for the rest of his or her life.

As I have found with many hundreds of patients, it may now be very difficult to get the balance of replacement therapy right, since for reasons not entirely clear, problems arise with the uptake of the synthetic thyroxine (we know the other thyroid hormones will assuredly not be given) and the conversion T4 → T3 doesn't work as it should, and tissue uptake doesn't take place as it should. It would seem logical, having wrecked thyroid function, that if replacement is required it should be provided as close to natural thyroid hormone as possible.

What seems to happen, however, is that our unfortunate patient, having repeated blood tests, finds blood levels swinging about from one extreme to the other, as the physician constantly tries to get it right by altering the thyroxine doses. The patient, of course never feels really well, sometimes ever again.

The second 'ablative' approach we saw is thyroid surgery. Let it be said at once that growths or cysts in the thyroid must be treated by surgical removal or a drainage procedure, and a much enlarged thyroid which interferes with breathing or swallowing leaves no option. But partial thyroidectomy to reduce the amount of thyroid hormone forming tissue is a popular, if in some eyes, barbaric procedure. It is popular with surgeons if only because, their job done, they may then refer the patient back to the physician for subsequent management.

My view is that as a procedure it should be the last resort only; and not as is so often and regrettably the case, almost the first option. Apart from all the normal objections to surgery, and a lasting reminder from the scar that one has had one's throat cut, the objection has to be the same as with 'nuking'; however can one make a good enough guess to get it right? Well, usually it isn't possible. Too little means the surgery may have to be done again, or suppressant drugs continued with; too much, and one falls back on thyroxine replacement. Sometimes the abused thyroid tissue may recover some function, so that the result of an over-enthusiastic surgical removal may in time largely correct itself. But many patients who have passed through my surgery doors have found themselves under-active sooner or later. Once again the patient is obliged to join the seesaw of more or less replacement therapy ever after, being told that they are perfectly well – *whatever* they say – since the blood tests show they are.

Inevitably I have seen many patients who are hypothyroid in consequence of this treatment. They are told that thyroxine will solve all their problems resulting from now being hypothyroid. Sometimes, sometimes, it does. But it doesn't do any such thing for a very large number of people. The thyroid produces, as we saw, T4, T3, T2, T1 and calcitonin (and possibly another hormone suspected by Broda Barnes) – this is how it works. Perhaps someone can tell me how one of the hormones, a synthetic precursor hormone, can do as well as the natural product. Well, largely I find it can't, and doesn't.

I find many people never recapture their original health, in spite of the constant adjustments of dose; and moreover they often turn out to be suffering from symptoms and signs of low adrenal function. Getting them right can be very difficult, but a combination of adrenal support, often natural, together with thyroid support, can go a very long way to restoring normal health.

Chapter Four

When Things Go Wrong – Part 2

The Under-active Thyroid Gland

Let us look at four case histories: people whose entire lives, very nearly, have been seriously damaged, even wrecked, by having hypothyroidism undiagnosed or improperly treated.

Case One

Mrs T is 47. She ran into trouble at the early age of 11, when her periods, which had started early, were so bad that her doctor put her on the pill. She had always been troubled with frequent tonsillitis, although her tonsils were not removed until she was 28. During her early teenage years, thyroid tissue was found at the back of her tongue – 'the lingual thyroid'. All her thyroid tests were 'normal'.

Her periods steadily got worse and eventually she had a hysterectomy when she was 39. Soon after this, she started to get episodes of abdominal pain, which resulted in her gall bladder being removed as well. Needless to say, none of this helped very much and at 41 she really started to get symptoms. Chief among these, were visual fading, sweats, thrush and extreme fatigue. She now had severe pain in the lingual thyroid, although her thyroid tests were still normal. Nevertheless, within a few months it was decided to destroy her thyroid tissue and she was given radioactive iodine. Without her thyroid gland, she was now given thyroxine, but severe head pains made life a misery; and at the hospital it was felt that the scarred thyroid was causing nerve root pressure. A total thyroidectomy was therefore decided upon. The operation had all sorts of complications but she was eventually able to leave hospital. Her health now further declined and she was told it was due to her ovaries and that they must be removed; which they were and she had an HRT implant.

In spite of all this dramatic intervention she got worse: visual disturbances became more severe, she could barely walk, she gained weight, suffered from fluid retention and anxiety attacks. Thyroid tests now showed that there was too much thyroxine in the bloodstream (causing the anxiety attacks) so it was reduced. She became worse than ever; she was sleepy all the time; she couldn't walk, she was terribly cold and in constant pain.

Some of you reading this may at once hazard a guess as to what the problem was. She was severely hypothyroid, but she was unable to use the thyroxine. Too much and she was ill and toxic; too little and she became myxoedematous. All that we had to do was to switch her Thyroxine (T4) to Tertroxin (T3). Subsequently, she was found to respond better to the T3 manufactured in the USA, called Cytomel. She now enjoys an active life, free of her terrible symptoms. She runs a brisk and caring thyroid help group of her own and lectures and writes about thyroid illness.

As a postscript, her daughter began to suffer at 21, but on thyroid replacement she too has happily regained her normal health.

Case Two

Born some 45 years ago, Mrs W noticed while a teenager that she had marked neck enlargement (as had it seemed her aunt, who had a goitre, and had always taken iodine drops, in spite of which she was always very ill). She was extra tired, felt her eyes were rather strange and always seemed to have boils.

Things became more of a worry after her children were born, when she was 20 and 24. She was told she had postnatal depression and was given Valium and antidepressants, which she took for 3 years. Slowly her health declined. She gained weight, the tiredness got worse, her skin became dry, her periods and PMT became unbearable. Her neck enlargement was diagnosed as a goitre but repeated thyroid tests were normal.

Life was beset with personal problems and she lost her marriage; happily she remarried. Four years ago she had multiple tests for abdominal troubles, never diagnosed, and she became very nearly bedridden with terrible fatigue, deteriorating eyesight and memory loss.

When seen in my clinic, it was clear from her symptoms that her adrenal function was poor and she was hypothyroid. She made a satisfactory response to treatment, which included cortisone to provide adrenal support and Tertroxin. Unfortunately, by now her menstrual bleeding was so bad that she had to have a hysterectomy and had developed breast cysts. The hospital declared her thyroid and adrenal treatment dangerous and discontinued it. All the improvement was lost and she became increasingly unwell. She lost most of her hair and had to spend much of her life in bed. She was finally told by the hospital that she had ME and would have to live with her problems.

I saw her again some months later to find her really very poorly indeed, with adrenal and thyroid dysfunction. She was restarted on her cortisone and her T3. Happily she is now restored very nearly to normal health; she can do normal housework, look after her children and cook every meal. She says that the return of her life and health is a miracle.

Case Three

Mrs B was born in 1936. Her mother noticed, as she grew up during the war years, that she was unreasonably tired, but put it down to frequent visits to the air-raid shelter.

However, her tiredness grew worse; and when her periods started (rather late) at 14, they were very heavy and painful. She began to lose her hair, and noticed that she was also losing it over her body. She began to suffer from terrible migraines and had episodes, quite without cause, of depression. Although bright and intelligent, she had problems concentrating and became nervous and anxious in exams, returning unjustifiably poor results. She remained always tired. The doctor told her she had 'neurasthenia' and she had most unkindly by now been labelled a hypochondriac. She married when she was 25, but took 3 years to conceive her only daughter. The pregnancy was a nightmare, the birth worse.

As time went on, she was troubled with recurrent skin problems, eczema, arthritis and weight gain. She developed diabetes, high blood pressure and anxiety attacks, with her permanent exhaustion overlying everything. She had had multiple tests for under-active thyroid, but they always came back 'normal' and the diagnosis was dismissed by two top thyroid specialists (who shall be nameless). All said that she was psychiatrically disturbed, except the consultant psychiatrist, who actually listened to her; he said that she was perfectly stable and there was physical illness behind her trouble.

When seen in my clinic some years ago now, it was clear that this lady had been hypothyroid all her life. She had done a lot of personal research and she knew it as well as I did. She was started on desiccated thyroid, and continues to take it to this day. Though late in life, she regained her energy and natural good humour and her other symptoms have slowly lifted. Thankful for her recovery, she started a thyroid help and support group and pointed many hundreds of people in the direction of full recovery.

Case Four

Mrs B was born in 1958. Although she was a normal teenager, she was always exhausted, and going to bed at 6 pm was not unusual for her at all. She was always tired and un-refreshed in the morning and had to fight to get up and go to work. By the age of 21 she began to notice some stiffness of her upper body, and a consultant neurologist diagnosed a mild form of muscular dystrophy. There was no family history of this – muscular dystrophy is very much inherited – but her mother and grandfather had thyroid illness.

During the next 15 years her general health deteriorated, and she became unable to walk anywhere, except about the house; although the muscular problem had altered little. The exhaustion became crippling; she was always ill and became depressed and anxious. She conceived when she was 37, but lost the baby and there was further deterioration in her general health. She could now barely walk at all without losing her balance. Next year she conceived and had her baby by caesarean section. She felt worse than ever and muscle wastage became evident. Her thyroid tests showed a T4 of 11.2, which was low, and a TSH of 5.1, which was clearly high, but she was told that they were perfectly all right. (See the TSH chart at the end of Chapter Nineteen.)

She sought private advice and was started on desiccated thyroid with limited improvement. It became clear that her adrenal glands were weakened and the T4 → T3 conversion was not working properly. Providing her with Prednisolone (a synthetic form of cortisone, one of the chief adrenal hormones) and T3 made a dramatic difference, and although she still occasionally has off days, her whole life has dramatically improved for the better, the muscle weakness continues to improve, she can walk anywhere she wants and can now look after her family and enjoy her great hobby, working in the garden.

* * *

We now come to understanding the under-active thyroid. Understanding is certainly the right word since many doctors have only the haziest idea of what it is all about, and many endocrinologists who claim to know, have more often than not actually got it wrong, following comfortable but distorted precepts considered correct by establishment medicine.

One point I want to make at once, is that hypothyroidism is getting more common.[1] A celebrated physician, Dr Starr, in 1920, reckoned that about 10% of the population was affected. In the late 1940s, Dr Broda Barnes revised this to 20%; by 1976 he had upped it again to 30%. Dr Jacques Hertoghe in the mid 1990s, even suggested nearly 80%.

Why this Increase?

One good reason is that hypothyroid children at the turn of the 20th century, with their faulty immune response, and the non-availability of vaccines and antibiotics, were simply lost. They did not live to pass on their faulty genes. Now, of course, medical science saves them. As they grow up, they are attracted to low thyroid partners (who, like themselves, would rather sit around than rush about) and so pass on the low thyroid genes. Two or three generations of this… and where are you?

Another good reason is that our environment with its toxins, heavy metals, and heaven knows what else besides attacking our thyroids, gives us no chance to escape.

There is of course the question of diagnosis. For reasons which are really not obvious, doctors would prefer to diagnose depressive illness, CFS/ME, gynae problems, old age or just plain hypochondria, instead of the obvious illness, staring them in the face all the time.

The level of circulating thyroid hormone, and the system's response to it, may be downgraded as a result of quite a large number of factors, and – this is important – it may be lowered by a few per cent only or one hundred per cent. The symptoms, and degree of illness, must therefore be related to the degree of loss. So how ill you are depends on how much loss there is, for how long it has been going on, and the degree of damage being done to all the systems and biological mechanisms of the body as a whole – which, of course, is everything, since all your tissues require thyroid hormone to work properly. No one, therefore, is affected in quite the same way, and it is all too easy to miss the diagnosis in the early stages because all the standard symptoms and signs are not present. As an example, consider someone in their sixties. Hair is thinning, skin a bit coarse, they are depressed a lot of the time. What is their doctor likely to say? "Well, dear, it's your age – what can you expect?".… "Next, please."

Chances are, the doctor is missing early thyroid deficiency. Even if you pointed a gun at him and asked for a blood test, it is more than likely to come back normal, or slightly down – 'nothing to worry about'. You would then be read a lecture about wicked and evil thyroid doctors who have taken it upon themselves to treat patients (thus taking advantage of their emotional state); hypochondriacal illness; getting into bad ways – such as thinking for yourself and standing your ground; or, infinitely worse, self-treating, thereby placing yourself in the terrible danger of getting better…

All right. Let's get down to it. What happens to make the thyroid processes fail?

We'll list the causes.

1) ***Failure of control*** (as with the over-active thyroid) from the pituitary gland. We call this secondary hypothyroidism – that is, not due to the thyroid itself, but a production failure due to not being told what to do. Failure of the hypothalamus to produce TRH adequately is tertiary hypothyroidism. Incidentally both may result in low TSH in established hypothyroidism.

2) ***Primary failure***. This is when the thyroid tissue itself does not work properly for a variety of reasons, which I will detail in a moment.

3) ***Conversion failure***. You will remember that the thyroxine has to be turned into tri-iodothyronine (the T4 $\rightarrow$ T3 reaction). This may not work properly.

4) ***Receptor uptake failure***. Every cell has 'receptors' where the thyroid hormone passes into the cell. These may be resistant and take up less than they should.

5) ***Adrenal insufficiency***. Damaged or overworked adrenal glands will work less well than normally and a lowered production of cortisol and DHEA from unresponsive adrenals will affect thyroid production, conversion and

receptor uptake. As we shall see, adrenal insufficiency produces a number of symptoms of its own, further complicating the whole picture.

We can deal with the control failure problem pretty easily, since everything said about control failure in the over-active thyroid earlier applies here in reverse. A reduced production of TRH from the hypothalamus will in turn induce a reduced amount of TSH. We saw that the brain influences the TRH in response to external factors (like cold, or a major life crisis), a general running down of the body as a whole such as illness, general debility or age, and by monitoring the circulatory thyroid hormone present in the bloodstream at that time. Clearly, finely balanced as this mechanism is, it is not difficult to see how it can go out of kilter without too much provocation, temporarily or over longer periods of time. This is called tertiary hypothyroidism. The same applies to pituitary function; the output of TSH may drop as a result, for example from a tumour within it, or nearby, which, far from making extra hormone (as in hyperthyroidism), may compress the hormone producing tissue and damage it and its hormone production. This is secondary hypothyroidism, and a particularly important example of this occurs in something called Sheehan's syndrome, when the pituitary becomes seriously damaged by failure of the blood supply within itself. The commonest cause is haemorrhaging following childbirth, when the mother suffers a major postnatal haemorrhage, although any major traumatic blood loss can do the same thing.

For reasons not always clear, the TSH receptors may not respond properly to the TRH and under-produce TSH, with obvious reduction therefore of thyroid hormones. These problems are not easy to correct in themselves but clinically may not cause undue difficulty, since adjustments to thyroid replacement may be all that is necessary (having excluded sinister causes, which will have brought with them other symptoms and which would point to the need for further investigations).

Primary Thyroid Failure

We come now to primary thyroid failure, which is by far the commonest cause of thyroid deficiency. And here there is a whole list of possible causes.

Genetic

The thyroid gland may not develop properly *in utero* (that is in the womb) and the baby is born with the thyroid inactive or only partially active. The baby has a protuberant abdomen and a greatly enlarged tongue, muscle weakness with marked loss of muscle tone, and is a true example of a cretin. The bridge of the nose is flattened and all bony development is delayed. While the latter is obvious to clinicians in charge of the baby, lesser degrees of hypothyroidism in the newborn and infancy may go unnoticed in spite of a blood test. The growth parameters don't work out properly; the baby may be a bad feeder and fail to thrive, it may sleep all the time. Oddly enough, the hyperactive child may sometimes also be hypothyroid. One of the most severely hypothyroid children that I saw in my surgery, was a girl 3 years old, thin as a rake, cold as ice, and with the activity of a cartoon Tasmanian devil. Everything was cast to the floor in a sort of blur, the mother beyond despair. She reverted to normal within 2 or 3 months of treatment.

To miss lesser degrees of hypothyroidism in children is a major disaster, because the child can never achieve its full potential. It will be intellectually or emotionally affected and may find itself labelled with a diagnosis of autism. The poor achiever at school is a very likely candidate, and it may not be revealed by blood tests. Attention deficit hyperactivity disorder (ADHD) is another aspect of the problem; some of these children are actually hypothyroid but are not diagnosed. The conventional treatment consists of stimulating brain activity by the use of amphetamine-like stimulants; restoring brain activity to normal by bringing thyroid function back online, obviously makes far better sense.

Failure to make the diagnosis will ruin someone's life.

The thyroid may be genetically programmed to fail during adult life. A common time is puberty, or the menarche (that is, when periods begin) or after the strain of pregnancy or a major life event. In fact, failure slowly occurs during the ageing process, but obviously at genetically programmed rates. Loss of thyroid activity is part of ageing anyway; and in the prematurely aged, loss of thyroid activity must be looked for. This has been called 'the thyropause'; but it is not usually a sudden event but a progressive and insidious one.

Excess iron (haemochromatosis) is another problem that has recently been receiving recognition. Haemochromatosis is a genetic disorder which allows absorption of too much iron from an ordinary diet. This excess iron is then deposited all over the body and causes damage to the liver, pancreas, heart, endocrine glands and joints. It is easily detected by a simple blood test and a check on the amount of iron (serum ferritin) in the blood. Although this is quite uncommon, it should be looked for since the treatment is so simple; the patient has to be bled monthly (just like they used to do in the old days).

The Environment

In this instance we are going to consider deficiencies and toxins. The deficiency most of us know about is that of iodine, which as we saw earlier, is the vital part of the molecule of the thyroid hormones. Certain soils have iodine naturally, and certain soils don't. As one source of iodine is fish, deficiency is more likely to be found in inland areas, as in the mountains of central Europe, and in the United

Kingdom in the Peak District. The deficiency causes enlargement of the thyroid, commonly called in England, 'Derbyshire Neck', when it increases in size to make up for the deficiency. The widespread use of less natural foods and the iodinization of salt have made this uncommon today; and iodine supplements for thyroid conditions are not only usually unnecessary but may be actively harmful. Too much iodine may actually suppress thyroid hormone production. But read a bit more about this in Chapter Seven.

Another deficiency of some importance is that of the element selenium. This shouldn't occur in balanced diets, but may occur with generally low quality diets in certain countries and social groups. Selenium is vital to the 5'-deiodinase enzymes that transform T4 into T3. It is a good idea to include this in any supplementation for a healthy thyroid. Other minerals have to be considered also: calcium, zinc, magnesium, manganese, boron, iron. The tyrosine of course comes from protein in our food – and poor, low protein diets will mean deficiency.

There are a number of environmental poisons which should trouble us more than deficiencies. In these I want to include the halogens bromine, chlorine and fluorine, and the heavy metals (some of which unfortunately are nowadays found in fish) as for example mercury, cadmium and lead.[2, 3, 4]

Mercury is extraordinarily toxic, and we are exposed to it from dental amalgam and as a preservative in vaccinations. It has been linked to an increasing incidence of autism.[5] The 5'-deiodinase enzymes which oversee the conversion of T4 $\rightarrow$ T3 are dependent on there being enough selenium. Selenium can be antagonised by mercury, which is one way mercury acts as a poison. This brings us to the question of dental amalgam, which is a worrying and controversial problem. In Appendix A, I have gone into this in some detail. If you think your dental amalgams may be a problem, discuss the issue carefully with your dentist.

We should also include in this list high dosage cortisones given for asthma or rheumatoid arthritis, for example. The list of industrial poisons is lengthy indeed, but I particularly want to mention dioxins and PCBs (polychlorinated biphenols), which are absorbed by fatty tissues and may remain in the body for many years.

Dioxins are polychlorinated dibenzo-p-dioxin and polychlorinated dibenzofuran. Both dioxins and PCBs are potentially serious problems for our health generally, and the thyroid in particular. These compounds have many industrial uses, and are used in a number of substances including pesticides and paint. They are liver poisons, interfere with reproductive processes, the immune system and suppress iodine uptake by the thyroid and its processing into the thyroid hormones.

You won't be surprised to hear that our old favourites, tea and coffee have a depressant effect on thyroid function as does tobacco and alcohol, certainly in excess; although I expect you didn't know that tea contains more natural fluoride than almost any other plant since it only grows successfully in fluoride rich soil.

The Brassica family, cabbages, sprouts, turnips and so on, produce thiouracil which as we saw earlier in purified form is used medically in the suppression of thyroid function. Much of the possible damage may be avoided by proper cooking. I am not saying you must give them up, just don't overdo them. Cassava root in semi-tropical countries has a similar effect.

Then there is a pretty substantial list of drugs whose side effects include suppression of thyroid function. One such is lithium, widely used in the treatment of bipolar mood disorder. Amiodarone, used in the control of heart arrhythmias, is another example, and barbiturates and aspirin are others. Any drug taken to excess may cause a degree of thyroid suppression since the biological mechanisms of the thyroid are really quite easily upset. In our polluted environment we are at constant risk. Some authorities have expressed concerns about the effects of electromagnetic fields to which we are now relentlessly exposed; and I can think of several patients whose troubles began when they moved to live near electric power lines. The fact is that there is almost nowhere in our houses which is free of equipment creating electromagnetic fields, and televisions, PCs and mobile phones have fallen under suspicion.

Exceptionally worrying among all these is the element *fluorine*. Some years ago fluoride salts were used in the control of the over-active thyroid, since fluoride is a tissue poison. But in the rush to use fluoride salts in so many modern chemicals and chemical processes, particularly fluorinated hydrocarbons, their toxic effect on the thyroid seems to have been forgotten. Worse still, the questionable use of fluoride in toothpastes means that we are all exposed to it, whether we like it or not. Some authorities have claimed that in carefully controlled amounts, it may assist in the prevention of dental decay; but as an enzyme poison it is doing untold damage to our thyroids. We'd do far better to eat less sugar and carbohydrate and clean our teeth with old-fashioned dental pastes without fluoride.

As if this wasn't enough, we now have it in our water supplies. Mercifully, not all water companies add it to our water (at present only 10% of the UK), in spite of well meaning but desperately misinformed pressures from a number of health authorities. Government attempts to enforce fluoridation of water should be fought against at all costs. Surely it makes sense to err on the side of caution?

The fluoride salts used are waste products from manufacturing processes and are cheap and plentiful, and I'm very sorry to say are shovelled into the water with poor regard for measured amounts. They aim for 1 or 2 or even 3 parts per million of fluoride to water but chemical testing has shown that much higher levels than this are by no means uncommon. Many people living in fluoridated catchment areas are exposed on a daily basis to levels of fluoride toxic to other body systems as well as the thyroid. I believe the increasing incidence of hypothyroidism is a major consequence of this, and the effect on the Gq/11 proteins is closely related to the increasing incidence of autism.

Perhaps even more worrying are the results of studies recently published in China. Comparing the Intelligence Quotient (IQ) of two groups of people from separate villages, one with 4 times more fluoride in the water than the other, it was found that there was very marked lowering of IQ scores in the higher fluoride group.[6]

Research in the USA as far back as 1944 (the Manhattan Project) showed that fluoride is a powerful central nervous system toxin. In 1995 and 1998 Dr Mullenix's research[7,8] showed that fluoride accumulates progressively in brain tissue, notably in that part of the brain called the hippocampus. Fluoride was also found to be associated with behavioural problems. Further evidence has shown that fluoride acts as an enzyme poison, affecting many enzymes within the body.[9,10] It was found that fluoride can be ingested at any time of life to wreak its damaging effects; but of great concern was the effect found in utero on brain development. Even very small amounts were shown to have an effect on the development of intelligence.[11,12]

The Gq/11 Connection

The effectiveness within the cells themselves of thyroid hormone, and we're now talking about liothyronine (T3), in raising the metabolic activity of the cell, is governed by substances which switch the process on, or switch it off. The alpha-adrenergic receptors are one such, and the enzyme phosphodiesterase is another. But of crucial importance are the G1 proteins, of which for thyroid receptors there are four, two to switch on and two to switch off. The chief and most important switcher off is the one called Gq/11.

The object of the Gq/11 especially is to inhibit or slow down the activity of T3 in stimulating cellular metabolism. If blood thyroid hormones are low, this is picked up by the hypothalamus and it responds by producing TRH, which now is passed to the pituitary to stimulate it to produce more TSH. TSH stimulates the thyroid to produce T4 & T3, but the T3 stimulates the production of Gq/11, which reduces the activity of T3 in the cell until blood levels have normalised. This is all very well and good unless there is, for some reason, an abnormal and exaggerated over-activity of Gq/11. This, it turns out, can happen under the influence of fluoride compounds, and silica, beryllium and aluminium; the result is that the metabolic activity of the cell is wrongly reduced.

It gets worse. Some fluoride compounds actually prevent the TRH – from the hypothalamus – binding to the pituitary cells which make the TSH. Consequently, the circulating TSH drops even though (due to low thyroid levels) it should be high. This of course means the TSH blood test may be quite wrong. So we have two really awful problems to worry about. One is that the Gq/11 proteins in our modern polluted environment may overwork and shut down thyroid activity – thus reducing metabolism – and the other is that if this does happen, blood tests may not show it, especially the widely used TSH test.

Unfortunately, we cannot even leave it there. We noted that these Gq/11 proteins are over-activated by the presence of fluoride, and that fluoride can also work to reduce TSH output; but fluoride has not finished its evil work yet. Fluoride can actually diplace the iodine in thyroid compounds, which means those with fluoride in their makeup don't work, although blood tests will show no sign of this, since being halogens the chemical response is the same. And if that wasn't enough, the conversion of T4 $\rightarrow$ T3 can also be interfered with. What happens here is that the 5'-deiodinase enzymes are targeted and reverse T3 is manufactured at the expense of normal T3, which as you will recall is biologically inactive, promoting a hypothyroid state.

There are a number of scientists, together with the National Pure Water Association, who have expressed their deep concerns to the powers that be about the risk of adding fluoride to water supplies. And even though attention has been drawn to the situation, far too many people in this country alone have no choice in the matter. I recommend most earnestly that you drink bottled fluoride-free water or filter your water. Use fluoride-free toothpaste and violently oppose any medical, dental or nursing suggestion that you should have drops or tablets of fluoride as a supplement. Fluoride is bad, bad news; its effect is slow and insidious but damaging and may be permanent. Of deep concern is recent evidence that it may be linked to autism, as is mercury. We cannot go on taking the risk. You might care to compile a list for yourself of the number of products in your home using fluorinated hydrocarbons.

We may be unable to do very much to avoid the environment damaging our thyroid, but we should know about it and at least lessen where we can the many different possible factors which, put together, may be significant.

Autoimmune Disease

The most common of these we have already mentioned – autoimmune thyroiditis or Hashimoto's disease. For an illness first described in Japan in 1912 it is remarkably common in the western world, and I rather think, more common as time passes.[13] The underlying problem is an autoimmune reaction by the system, where the defence mechanisms which produce antibodies to combat bacterial and foreign body invasion, turn in on the body itself.

A word here about autoimmune disease. We constantly have to fight against foreign invaders which challenge our health and the integrity of our system. Broadly speaking, two groups of white cells in the blood arm themselves for this role. One such battalion is formed from the T cells. T cell forces are divided into the helper cells, and the killer cells. The helper cells are the reconnaissance party, and seek out and identify the foreign invaders – like a bacterium or flu germ, for example – and then call up reinforcements. These are the killer cells, which appear with swords unsheathed and deal with the invaders. They have a memory for the intruding enemy, and next time there is an attempted invasion they are ready for all comers. (That's why you don't get mumps twice.)

The second battalion comprises the B cells. These too seek out the foreign protein and synthesise a protein antibody, called an immunoglobulin, specific for the invader, which is then immobilised. It is then eaten... The cannibals are also white cells called phagocytes.

This process can go wrong; sometimes the 'invader' isn't really an invader at all, but part of the system quietly going about its business, but which gets attacked just the same, or overwhelmed by an excessive overreaction by both T and B cells. The result is that a normal tissue becomes invaded and progressively destroyed. Rheumatoid arthritis, temporal arteritis, systemic sclerosis, systemic lupus erythematosus (SLE), are examples of this happening; these are called collagen disorders. In fact, there is a group of disorders called **autoimmune polyglandular syndromes (APS)**. There are three chief syndromes; and one, APS II, is a real problem, since the autoimmune process attacks not just the thyroid, but the adrenals and other glands and tissues as well. When the thyroid and adrenal glands alone are attacked it is called **Schmidt's syndrome**.

In **Hashimoto's disease**, antibodies to the thyroid are launched and latch onto receptors within the thyroid, and may switch them on to promote over-activity. So there may be a period of months, or even years, where the thyroid is over-active. But sooner or later, this situation goes into reverse and the thyroid starts to slow down. The initial over-active phase may not occur, or is not noticed. In any laboratory workup for thyroid illness, antibodies are, or should be, checked for. Their presence, however, will little affect the ultimate treatment. The evolution of autoimmune thyroiditis is one of progressive deterioration of thyroid function; the thyroid may slowly enlarge or shrink, its hormone production lessening as time goes by. Hashimoto's disease is a slow inexorable deterioration, and it may take years for the diagnosis to be made. We'll note, just in passing, two other forms of degenerative thyroid disease: de Quervain's thyroiditis and Reidel's thyroiditis. Both are uncommon, but result in progressive loss of thyroid function.

I should mention that there are acute forms of thyroiditis, or thyroid inflammation which, often virally induced, may flare up overnight. The patient may be quite ill and suffer from an acute over-active phase, which may pass in a relatively short time, and normality return. The gland itself becomes enlarged and painful with biochemical evidence of over-activity apparent. Most of these episodes pass, but can relapse, or progress to under-activity.

Glandular Fever

Commonly also called infectious mononucleosis, this is a viral condition affecting the whole body caused by the Epstein-Barr virus, cytomegalovirus, Coxsackie virus and others. The patient develops a frightful sore throat, enlarged tonsils often covered in white exudates, massively enlarged neck glands sometimes with involvement of other lymphatic glands throughout the body, a high fever, and a general illness which may last several days, or several weeks causing great debility. There is often no treatment that can be of any help – antibiotics usually don't work at all – although a short sharp course of cortisone has been found to limit the progression of the illness. Whilst in most cases the illness runs its course, the patient is often quite unwell for weeks or months afterwards and there may be episodes of relapse. What, however, is not realised by doctors is that in a proportion of cases the causative virus holes up in the colloid (hormone producing) tissue of the thyroid and progressively damages it.[14,15] It may not be apparent for many months or even years, since the thyroid may be able to compensate with tissue so far undamaged; but as time goes on, the symptoms of thyroid under-activity, usually put down to something else, may slowly begin to show themselves. In my clinic about 30% of thyroid patients give a history of glandular fever some time before they became ill with their thyroid problem.

Major Trauma

This means bad accidents primarily but we can include devastating life events. It seems that the system becomes so damaged that things never quite restore themselves. The thyroid may suffer directly in this way, but also indirectly from control failure as we mentioned above; or the adrenal system may be damaged in such a way as to interfere with thyroid hormone processing and uptake. The story runs that the patient was perfectly well until the road accident; the physical damage heals but the patient loses energy and drive, puts on weight and is really never the same again.

Thyroid Trauma

This means that the thyroid gland, exposed as it is, may be the subject of damage from the outside. One obvious example here is whiplash injury. Something like 30% of people who suffered whiplash injury have been found to develop hypothyroidism. Another obvious one is somebody getting you by the throat; and over vigorous examination has also been cited as a cause. Stretching the neck, as for example, banging your chin on the dashboard in a car crash, is another one.[16]

In a further study it was found that a proportion of patients, who had previous neck injury apparently developed fibromyalgia,[17] (partially, I would suggest, as a consequence of thyroid failure).

Surgery

In much the same way as major trauma, there may be a lasting effect on the body from surgery. There are three operations which seem to affect people most especially. Cholecystectomy is one, where the gall bladder is removed for gallstones. It is the ladies who pull the short straw in this one; it's uncommon in gentlemen. Another quite notorious operation is hysterectomy. Rare indeed is the lady who finds that weight gain and exhaustion do not begin after her surgery. Her weight gain will be put down to overeating 'to comfort herself for her lost fertility'. (I'm serious – doctors do actually come up with this hoary old chestnut.) It seems that there is some kind of hormonal dialogue between the womb and the thyroid, and any intrusion or disturbance of this balance may affect thyroid function. Even sterilisation, sometimes a simple D & C or termination of pregnancy may have this effect.

The other surgical intervention, which is far too common, is that of tonsillectomy. However necessary, this is a pretty barbaric operation, and massive primary or secondary haemorrhage may occur. There is a shared blood supply between the tonsils and the thyroid gland and the upshot of the surgery can be that the blood supply to the thyroid is damaged, which will mean a deterioration in thyroid function. At first this may be compensated for but as time wears on thyroid output falls slowly. I have seen many patients, often young adults, who have had their tonsillectomy in their teens with all the sequelae of low thyroid output developing within a year or so.

Pregnancy

Pregnancy is a frightful onslaught on the female metabolism from which most of the ladies manage to recover. During pregnancy, the metabolism usually runs a bit more briskly; but after childbirth there may be a problem re-attaining normal balance. Commonly there is a temporary slow-down – although the reverse can happen – which puts itself right in a month or so. It is traumatic pregnancy, where things haven't gone right in various ways (for example a caesarean section), which is most likely to create an end result where thyroid function may not recover. Heavy blood loss, as from a retained placenta, may be especially damaging.

Multiple pregnancy is a variation on traumatic pregnancy, as is having several pregnancies within a short time. Perhaps after the third or fourth little visitor, mum remains exhausted and cannot control her weight. Since mothers are expected to feel like this with several children, she may well make nothing of it and put it all down to life in general; and the doctor has several ready made excuses for not really listening. Postnatal depression is actually very commonly due to deficient thyroid function but thyroid as a cause is unlikely to be thought of; and if it is, the blood tests may be unrevealing. Another complication of childbirth is postpartum thyroiditis. This is inflammation of the thyroid gland, usually occurring 4-12 months after childbirth, with phases of both hyperthyroidism and hypothyroidism, and it usually lasts between 2 and 4 months. While low thyroid function – and consequent postnatal depression – may well be self-correcting, it may not be…

One last word. Some of you may have heard of the **sick euthyroid syndrome** and wondered what it was. We shall come across the term in Chapter Eleven on Reverse T3 and Doctor Wilson. What sick euthyroid means when used by your

NHS doctor, is that all tests are abnormal; but the patient is fine. This causes a management problem, since the doctor doesn't know whether to treat the patient, who makes no complaint, or not. In fact what happens is that sooner or later, and sometimes sooner, the patient does eventually become ill and will need treatment.

Actually, what sick euthyroid can also mean, and is more commonly seen but rarely acted upon, is that the tests are all normal, but the patient is obviously ill. This we may call euthyroid hypometabolism. The T4 seems normal and so does the T3 and the TSH. What happens is that the T4 doesn't convert properly into T3; and some turns into the inactive reverse T3, which blocks the receptor sites. There is apparently enough T3 but the actual tissue levels are low. This situation may occur with growth hormone deficiency, nutritional failures and low adrenal function.

Having had a careful look at how and why the thyroid becomes under-active, we must now see what it does to us when this happens.

Chapter Five

Hypothyroidism – The Symptoms

All illnesses are considered in a routine way to enable them to be properly diagnosed and treated; and hypothyroidism is no exception. The doctor listens to the symptoms and family history of illness; then examines for the signs – at this point taking the patient's temperature is invaluable since the consequent blessed silence enables him to think it all out in peace and quiet while wondering what on earth is going on – after which the diagnosis is made. Various tests may be needed to confirm this, after which treatment or 'management' is decided upon. There is many a slip twixt cup and lip, and everything you are reading is to make sure that there are *no* slips. So we come to the symptoms.

Let it be said at once, that there may be so many symptoms that if the patient doesn't think he or she is a hypochondriac, the doctor certainly may. As I said earlier, low thyroid can affect the working of any or all bodily systems. The particular mix of symptoms will depend on the person themselves, the severity of the deficiency and the length of time it's all been going on. But there are symptoms which invariably occur and several of them together should arouse a high index of suspicion. Some of these you have come across already, but I will go through them again. I make no apology for the length of the list and I don't want you skipping them. (I've made a more complete list in Appendix B.) Nor do I want it said that the trawl is so wide that you can include anything; many symptoms of course can have other causes. It is the way they all link up, followed by putting together the strands of evidence from the signs and tests that make the diagnosis clear and definite. Here we go...

Weight Gain

Very nearly the most common is weight gain. The patient, unable to utilise calories properly and perhaps too tired to exercise, finds that the unused calories turn to fat. Most people with an under-active thyroid are overweight and look puffy and fluidy. This in spite of sometimes rigorous dieting which usually fails and may actually make everything worse as time passes. It does also happen, however, that the thyroid failure may affect absorption from digestion, and this may cause weight loss and vitamin and mineral deficiencies. This is much more likely if the adrenal axis has been affected.

The problem with dieting if your thyroid is low is that the low food intake lowers the metabolism further, so you can finish up on a hiding to nothing; and are in great trouble if, in despair, you give up the dieting, having by then caused further lowering of the metabolism. Anything you lost you put back – and more besides. Incidentally all dieting can do this, which is why you have to come out of the dieting gradually, to allow the increased calorie intake to speed the metabolism back up.

Lowered Body Temperature

A low body temperature is most frequently complained of. You easily feel the cold, and go around with extra jumpers turning up the heating to the annoyance of other less chilly mortals. People say how cold your hands are, and you may look cold, white or blue for little cause. You come into your own only on the beach in Tenerife. The extra warmth in the environment means that your metabolism doesn't have to work so hard to maintain your body temperature. So you feel better altogether, your lowered thyroid output now sufficient for your needs. It may have been noted that, should your temperature be taken, it is always lower than anybody else's, and a sharp dose of flu merely brings your temperature to normal. Another symptom of this is that some people complain of shivering in the late afternoon, or waking at night extra cold.

Oddly enough, the hypothyroid state may affect your ability to regulate your body temperature: you don't sweat much and may be greatly troubled by excess heat as well as the cold. In summary, hypothyroidism causes intolerance of both cold and heat.

Lack of Energy

Probably the bitterest complaints centre around lack of energy; the sufferer is unnaturally tired with extreme muscle fatigue. You find you can't get up in the morning and drag yourself around for an hour or so before getting going. Or a terrible exhaustion may come upon you during the day; you doze off at your desk, or in the train, or watching the telly news. Just climbing the stairs at the station may cause exhaustion and dreadful muscle pain in your legs. The drive and vigour that once were yours seems to have evaporated: your get up and go has got up and gone. You have to force yourself to do things by an effort of will. Strong-minded people go to the gym, and the leaping about temporarily restores their energy levels – which then slowly run down again the next day. However, if you completely crash after exercise, there is most likely an adrenal component to your illness, of which more later. A strong psychic drive *can* keep people going; but at the end of their day there is nothing left except a terrible weariness.

'I'm so tired doctor' – a pretty familiar opening remark, which may provoke this pretty standard response; 'of course you're tired – look at your age / work / children'. A general blood test may reveal little (perhaps a little anaemia and a raised cholesterol) and the thyroid tests turns out to be in the normal range. So you are properly wrong-footed. But your exhaustion, unrelieved by sleep, goes on and on ...

Fluid Retention

We're up to the fourth commonest hypothyroid symptom, and that is fluid retention. Actually this has two components. The first is fluid held in a chemical matrix with waste products of metabolism to form compounds called mucopolysaccharides. As time passes, instead of being excreted, these mucopolysaccharides accumulate in the tissues, causing a general puffiness, and thickness of the skin. This may be particularly obvious in the face and the legs, and gives its name to the old term for hypothyroidism: 'myxoedema'. Strictly speaking this term is now reserved for the more extreme, or terminal phase of thyroid dysfunction; lesser degrees we tend to call thyroid deficiency or thyroid dysfunction, or simply hypothyroidism. The important feature of myxoedema is that the fluid cannot be got rid of by the usual diuretics; it will slowly disappear only on replacement therapy for the missing thyroid hormone.

But in the same way that nothing really works properly in a hypothyroid state, the proper blood filtration and maintenance of normal fluid balance, which is the responsibility of the kidneys, doesn't work as it should, and facial puffiness, especially around the eyes – we call this periorbital oedema – and swelling of the ankles also becomes a problem. Unlike the oedema mentioned above, this second type of fluid retention comes and goes, and 'pits' on firm finger tipped pressure. This *will* respond to diuretics, like bendrofluazide or frusemide, but of course it comes back. This has a more sinister side: poor kidney function releases a hormone called renin, which is metabolised into another hormone called angiotensin, and this is the system's chemical way of putting up the blood pressure, the idea being to increase kidney filtration by forcing extra blood through them. I needn't remind you that blood pressure increase is a bad thing whichever way you look at it. And it gets worse, of course. How often do you think low thyroid is considered as a cause of hypertension? (Bearing in mind, as Broda Barnes clearly stated in his book *Hypothyroidism – The Unsuspected Illness*, that one in three or one in four people by mid-life may suffer from hypothyroidism, and the American Association of Clinical Endocrinologists says that 1 in 10 Americans suffer from thyroid disease.) The answer is almost never. I have to say, and say it very loudly indeed, that any patient with unexplained fluid retention and/or hypertension *must* be considered for hypothyroidism. Don't take anyone's word for it. You may have to do the considering yourself, and I'll show you as we go on, how you can.

Chronic Constipation

The next common symptom is chronic constipation. The general sluggishness of the system as a whole extends to the gut. Many people come to terms with this problem by regularly taking some sort of laxative on a long-term basis. The whole thing slows down, and the "transit" time, commonly between 12 and 24 hours between eating and opening of the bowel, may be doubled or trebled. Piles or painful defecation may be a corroborative symptom. Just occasionally, especially if there is malabsorption, as with adrenal weakness, diarrhoea may be a presenting symptom.

Women are more likely to admit to constipation; men, being more basic, as we know, tend to be regular on principle. Sometimes the constipation is really quite extreme; it may be a week between each bowel action. Haemorrhoids are a common result of this, and many people develop intractable thrush (candida). Treating this without getting the bowel going regularly is bound to fail. People perhaps don't always like to mention it but excessive flatulence can also be a very real problem.

Chapter Five

Nervous Disorders

We must now consider nervous disorders. Brain cells have more T3 receptors than any other tissues, which means that a proper uptake of thyroid hormone is essential for the brain cells to work properly. So we won't be surprised to hear that hypothyroidism can cause all sorts of nervous problems. Most common is depression. So many people get depressed, especially in middle life, and it is always possible to find reasons. The empty nest syndrome, job uncertainties, marital difficulties, failure in health and vigour; you name them. And it is so easy to treat – Prozac, and so many other antidepressants, may be given at the flourish of a pen – and doubtless many people improve. And few doctors will think that it may simply be due to thyroid deficiencies. I say to you now that one third to one half of depressed folk are suffering from unrecognised hypothyroidism.[1,2] Some are in psychiatric wards, and taking expensive and powerful psychotropic (mood altering) medication, with all the attendant risks of dependence and side effects. Prozac is an especially unfortunate choice, since its molecule contains fluoride – and therefore any improvement may be at the heavy price of worsening the underlying cause.

Here, I believe, is one great scandal of undiagnosed hypothyroidism. If you have been diagnosed as depressed (especially without good cause) read this book through; think about it, talk about it, get tests done if you can or evaluate yourself on the basis of symptoms and signs that we are now discussing; in particular read Chapter Nineteen. If you don't think about it, the diagnosis will be missed – you may be condemned to months or years of medication and a shadow existence. This last paragraph will go down very badly with many doctors and probably many psychiatrists. But you should be able, when you have finished reading these chapters, to make a valid diagnosis yourself. (This will go down even worse, because doctors don't like patients making up their own minds about anything medical. But you can, you can.)

Loss of Memory and Thinking Ability

One of the symptoms that upsets a hypothyroid sufferer almost more than anything, is the slow but inexorable loss of grasp. Always forgetting appointments, or names, or things planned to do. So many will admit to this if you ask – putting it down to age or overwork or worry or whatever; and they compensate by carrying a diary around with them. Everything gets written down. (I myself found that my ability to think straight, work things out, diagnose, prepare a treatment programme, became within 2 or 3 months of treatment so much easier. It was like someone turning on the lights.)

Speech slows down and there is a pause before they work out what they are saying. They may not perhaps notice it themselves, but others do. Alongside this loss of cognitive function, there may develop anxiety attacks, agoraphobia or claustrophobia or full-blown panic attacks. So it is really frightfully important to get the diagnosis right, because regular tranquillisers or antidepressants are really an admission of medical failure. Insomnia is a common complication of all of the above; and thyroid supplementation may, between 2 and 3 weeks, restore normal sleeping. You might have thought that it would wind you up and make insomnia worse, but it doesn't unless the dose is becoming too high. In all elderly patients losing their faculties, this is a desperately important physical cause that should be considered. (If they are hypothyroid, they improve, always.)

Arthralgia

Arthralgia is a very broad term, which basically means aches and pains, apparently in all your muscles and joints. In this we can include rheumatoid arthritis, osteoarthritis, systemic lupus erythematosus (SLE) and anything else which makes you creak and groan. Evidence is mounting – not, of course, much accepted by many doctors – that many of these apparently degenerative illnesses are the result of the immune system not working as it should. We cannot, and must not, blame these illnesses necessarily entirely on loss of thyroid function; but there are connections. If systems as important as the thyroid and the adrenals are slipping out of whack, so too will be the immune system. Another odd, but common symptom, is that of shooting pains – for no obvious cause – in the hands and feet or sometimes elsewhere.

Hypothyroidism does, however, have a direct role to play in causing pain and stiffness in muscles, ligaments and joints. And this is the result of the deposition I mentioned of mucopolysaccharides. These accumulate within the fibrous and connective tissues of joints and muscles and ligaments and interfere with their proper functioning. The result is aches and pains and stiffness. Anyone whose thyroid has started to fail will become troubled with rheumatics. But it is all reversible. As the thyroid status improves on treatment, the mucopolysaccharides slowly get removed and the muscles and joints free up. People complain of neck and shoulder pain; that they have a heavy head making it tiresome to keep the head upright.

Headaches

Intractable headaches can be a feature of hypothyroidism and hypoadrenalism. They are not improved by rest or relaxation, and have no obvious cause. It is not really clear why headache should be such a problem, but it may be related to the fluid retention increasing pressure within the brain. They get better on treatment.

Skin

Skin troubles with hypothyroidism are many and various. In general the skin is dry, coarse and thickened. Classically furunculosis and folliculitis are to be expected.

Sorry – boils and spots. An outbreak of either at the wrong time of one's life should arouse suspicion. But rashes, dermatitis and eczema may also start appearing for no good reason. The skin may be generally unhealthy looking, sallow and lack lustre. Not uncommonly, there may be a degree of yellow pigmentation of variable degree. This is due to the deposition in the skin of beta carotene, from vegetables primarily, since in hypothyroidism it may not be metabolised properly in the liver to vitamin A. Most commonly, the extra beta-carotene one may have been taking to ward off the symptoms of tiredness and exhaustion brought about by hypothyroidism, may well be another cause of excess carotene in the blood and skin.

Hair Loss

Thinning hair over the scalp is of course to be expected in gentlemen and it would not be easy to decide on a primary cause, but it may be more obvious in the ladies. The hair becomes fine and wispy and falls out constantly. It may be severe enough to be diagnosed as alopecia areata, where the hair loss is uneven and patchy, as opposed to alopecia totalis which, as you may imagine, may result in a general loss of hair; not just the scalp but elsewhere as in armpits and pubic region. It's an important and regularly seen symptom and may be the reason you first took yourself to the doctor. Patients may also complain both of loss of frontal hair and hair at the back of the head. Another classical symptom is loss of the outer third of the eyebrows, or loss of eyelashes – sometimes both.

Changes in the Voice

Another symptom which will distress the ladies is a deepening and hoarseness of the voice. This may or may not be associated with a feeling of discomfort in the throat when breathing or swallowing. In addition, an enlargement of the neck from the thyroid itself may become quite uncomfortable. This is of course, the goitre, which may be present in both over-active and under-active thyroid states. In practice, the thyroid tissue seems most commonly to shrink, and may be actually quite difficult to feel at all.

Poor Resistance to Infection

This may be a very important symptom, but not recognised as such. Upper respiratory tract infections (URTI) may show themselves as repeated coughs and colds, a tendency to catch anything that is going. With poor thyroid activity and nothing working as well as it should, we find the immune system is sluggish and slow in its response to infection. Delayed wound healing is another side to this. This applies also to urinary tract infections (UTI), which may be most persistent in the ladies, young and old, who become troubled with persistent and repeated cystitis and/or kidney infections. The bladder becomes irritable and causes unreasonable frequency. In children, enuresis (night wetting) is a common complaint. Any schoolgirl repeatedly troubled in this way should be considered for thyroid under-activity.

Atherosclerosis

You may wonder why I am leaving this crucially important aspect close to last. Problem is, you don't *get* symptoms of atherosclerosis until it is already there; and you get a rise in blood pressure and a chest tightness on exertion when it is nearly too late to do anything. This is why if your thyroid is failing the sooner you know about it the better. Your life is at stake.

We tend to think of atherosclerosis as 'hardening of the arteries' but it is not so much a hardening, as deposition of cholesterol within the lining of the arteries and consequent damage so that the arteries become narrowed. When this happens, as it now does with terrifying frequency to coronary arteries, aided and abetted by smoking, we have the epidemic and scourge of our time, coronary thrombosis with the risk of sudden death. Well, low thyroid function is a bigger cause of cholesterol build up in the blood than bad eating. We are told over and over again how we must reduce our cholesterol intake; we change the way we eat, and take expensive anti-cholesterol drugs to do this. Many of these drugs so freely prescribed and promoted by the drug companies have inherent dangers of their own, apart from their expense. Indeed, as recently as August 2001, Schatz, a professor of medicine at the University of Hawaii, published a disturbing paper which showed that reducing cholesterol to the levels now considered healthy, may actually have a reverse effect.[3] He went on to say that 'those with cholesterol levels widely assumed to be healthy had a roughly 35-40% greater chance of dying from any cause in the following 25 years'. And all the time it is low thyroid which bears a heavy (though doubtless not an exclusive) responsibility. Physicians are simply not aware how devastating low thyroid is in this respect.

Broda Barnes pointed out 40 years ago that vegetarian animals (like rabbits and sheep) who eat no meat or fat and have in consequence low levels of cholesterol in the blood in the normal healthy state, will experience a sustained rise in cholesterol if the thyroid is removed; and that if thyroid hormone is then administered, it drops again.[4] How is it that this knowledge has been forgotten for so many years? The test for cholesterol in patients with low thyroid always shows it to be elevated (cholesterol elevation used to be a measure of thyroid levels); and after treatment, it always goes down. But today the diagnosis is not made and the root cause not corrected.

In another study, over 30 years, Barnes[5] showed that if you keep your patients euthyroid (that is at normal thyroid levels) the incidence of coronary thrombosis dropped dramatically, even to vanishing point, the longer the patient was treated. He also showed that the incidence of breast cancer was similarly dramatically reduced. This study has been fully supported by Dr Derry, in Canada,[6] who researched the connection between the thyroid, iodine and breast cancer. (I refer to this in more detail in Chapter Seven.) Dr Derry fought a long and brave battle with the medical establishment in Canada to justify his use of thyroid treatment. The bottom line is that preventing and curing hypothyroidism will largely if not completely prevent coronary thrombosis and breast cancer. (The role thyroid plays in other cancers is yet to be researched, but since a healthy immune system is necessary to prevent cancer and a healthy immune system is dependent on the correct individual thyroid levels, there seems to be a very important place for further research.) These simple and proven facts are quite ignored by most doctors. Can you think of a bigger scandal than this? Is it really just coincidence that there is an increase of cancer and coronary disease and an increase in untreated thyroid disease?

While we are on the subject, the heart muscle is itself affected; it is weakened and enlarged, which causes poor contractility. This will cause breathlessness, angina and fluid retention. The rhythm of the heart may become disturbed and irregular.

People don't have to die. Just make sure your thyroid status is normal and if it isn't, treat it, whatever your doctor says.

Anaemia

Many people with hypothyroidism suffer from anaemia. This may be because of poor absorption of vitamin B_{12}, when abnormal size and shape of the red blood cells will confirm the diagnosis. Sometimes the anaemia is related to poor absorption of iron, or a constant loss of iron in women due to heavy and prolonged periods. For the bone marrow to manufacture new blood cells it needs to be at the right temperature. The generally low body temperature of hypothyroidism may mean a chronically low level of red cell production, that is, anaemia, which won't respond to vitamins or iron, but only to thyroid supplementation.

Loss of Libido

Sadly, loss of libido is a most common symptom which patients may not necessarily tell the doctor about. Especially common after childbirth due to the thyroid connection, it becomes a potent cause of troubles within the marriage. It responds well to thyroid supplementation.

Infertility

Infertility troubles so many couples. How many gynaecologists routinely and carefully check the thyroid? Very few I'm afraid. And yet low thyroid is one of the most common causes of infertility. Another very often seen result of low thyroid is repeated miscarriage for no obvious cause. And it's not just women; the fertility of their partners may be equally damaged. The usual story is that all tests are normal and so they may appear; but low thyroid may be there just the same.

Menstruation, Childbirth and Postnatal Depression

Thyroid dysfunction can have devastating effects on menstruation and childbirth. Looking first at **menstruation**: hypothyroidism will crucially affect the start of periods (the menarche). Oddly enough it can do it in two opposite ways. It can cause the menarche to start earlier than it should – 8, 9, or 10 years old – or much later than it should – 15, 16 or 17 years old, for example. Characteristically, the periods may be disorganised and irregular, and much too painful. It has been shown that low thyroid affects the way the other hormones (oestrogen and progesterone) which control the menstrual cycle, are produced. Herein lies the reason why some girls have such a hard time of it during the early years of menstruation. Any teenager with menstrual problems must have their oestrogen and progesterone checked several times during a cycle; and a careful assessment of thyroid function should be made.

Childbirth may be profoundly affected. Sometimes the general gearing up of the system may prop up a thyroid beginning to fail; typically the mother may feel really well and full of energy and drive – only to lose it soon after the birth of the baby. (The extra oestrogen and progesterone, as the result of the pregnancy, have the effect of releasing more thyroid hormones from the binding sites.) Sometimes, it doesn't work like that; and the pregnancy becomes a frightful trial with enormous weight gain, in spite of all care, which won't come off afterwards. The confinement may not be as normal and straightforward as with a mother with normal thyroid function, and there are usually complications of one sort or another. Sounds familiar? Well, read on.

If as a mother your thyroid is low, the baby may help you out. As the baby's thyroid develops, it may compensate for the lack in the mother's thyroid by producing extra thyroid of its own. (Much of the baby's thyroid hormone is in a different form, called reverse T3, which has very little biological activity. Nevertheless there may be more thyroid available than normal.) And here is something you were not expecting; thyroid can also act as a growth hormone in early life. It is needed in a greater or lesser degree in young animals; for example, if you give tadpoles thyroid hormone, they start turning much too early into very small frogs. In the womb the extra thyroid encourages growth in the baby. Any mother who produces a baby close to or over 9lb is likely to have one of two possible problems. (Assuming dad isn't enormous of course.) She may have early diabetes, or she may have a thyroid which is beginning to fail. The diabetes is easily decided by checking the urine and blood; the thyroid is not so easy, unless checked in the ways I shall be telling you about.

Postnatal Depression. Lots of mothers have a spell after having the baby of being depressed. And the physical and emotional strain is more than likely to need time to settle down. But the thyroid can go out of kilter in either way. Over-activity is usually brief and self-correcting and clinically obvious, so it gets noticed.

Under-activity may be much less obvious and since it often doesn't show on blood tests, doesn't get diagnosed. The depression and tiredness drags on and on ('Why doesn't she pull herself together?') and weight doesn't get lost or starts to increase. No case of postnatal depression should ever be treated without careful consideration of possible thyroid involvement. In very many cases it will indeed be found. Other causes are thought to be related to the sudden loss of progesterone, which is running at high levels in pregnancy, or adrenal exhaustion from the stress of it all.

Other Symptoms

This list has seemed pretty endless. But, it isn't exhaustive. Hypothyroidism I often think of as the 'great pretender'. It can mimic almost any illness known to man, and some of the symptoms reported to me are often extraordinary. One such is hypoglycaemia (low blood sugar), which is often considered an illness in its own right; it isn't; it is caused by a control problem. Hypothyroidism may well be the underlying cause, as may also low adrenal function, and sometimes of course both. Other symptoms include visual disturbances, where there is loss of colour perception and the world becomes grey; there may even be hallucinations. There may also be reported breathlessness on quite minor exertion and even chest pain and palpitations. Nails may grow poorly and be subject to flaking. The patient may not only be visibly pale but there may be evidence of cyanosis (blueness) of the lips. Many people with low thyroid function develop Raynaud's phenomenon. Here on quite minor exposure of the hands or feet to cold, the circulation shuts down completely and the patient develops very cold white or blue hands. Surgery is often recommended for this condition but the answer is actually likely to be thyroid supplementation. Another quite common presentation of low thyroid can be carpal tunnel syndrome. Here the patient develops episodes of disabling pain in the wrists and hands. This too is usually dealt with by surgery but the chances are very high that hypothyroidism is the underlying cause. With Hashimoto's disease, one must also look out for the related autoimmune disorders, which may be: pernicious anaemia (low B_{12}), calcium deficiency due to low parathyroid hormone function, diabetes mellitus (Type I), Addison's disease, premature menopause and vitiligo (loss of pigmentation in the skin).

Although it could well be argued that anybody can have any of these symptoms, for any reason, the very number of them together with the signs found on examination, will lead the discerning physician to no other conclusion.

So now let us look at the signs.

Chapter Six

Hypothyroidism – The Signs

Signs are the things about a patient that a doctor looks for to help him make his diagnosis; that is to say the symptoms, and the family history of illness. For example, if 'I've got a sore throat doctor' is followed by the doctor observing that the patient has a raised temperature, and when he looks down the throat there are monstrous red tonsils, then the diagnosis is acute tonsillitis. This is basically how all illnesses are diagnosed and hypothyroidism is no exception. The experienced physician can make a diagnosis on his knowledge and experience, and this is what mostly happens.

However, there are illnesses more complicated, and more rare, which have several diagnostic possibilities, and so is done the 'blood test'. The problem with the blood test is that it is a bit like looking up the answers in the back, to save one the fag of thinking. Then there is the obligation to do a blood test, which has become fashionable and the done thing to do, even though it is probably not always necessary. This is the hospital specialist's approach and it is taken to an extreme in the USA (and pretty much so in the UK). All patients in the USA carry around with them a vast battery of test results (at huge expense) and the excellence, or otherwise, of the specialist is judged by the number of tests he orders. We find ourselves in the grip of a medico-technocracy. The blood test is god, and eventually takes over the diagnostic process. I deeply deplore this state of affairs, since I was taught and have never had any reason to doubt, that the best diagnostic weapons of all are the Mark I eyeball and the Mark I earhole. Look and listen. The other excellent lesson I learnt was that if the blood test doesn't bear out your diagnosis, believe in your own learning and experience.

In no branch of medicine is this more true than that of thyroid medicine. Since 1898 doctors have been diagnosing hypothyroidism, but in the last three or four decades medical dogma has come to say, *you cannot and must not make the diagnosis without THE BLOOD TEST*. There have been about 40 different tests for thyroid illness because not one has been found to be reliable. When I was first a doctor, a blood test called the plasma bound iodine (PBI) was becoming the rage. Only trouble was it kept finding perfectly normal patients hypothyroid and missing obviously sick people. Eventually, it was decided that iodine in the apparatus, and in the air of the laboratory itself, was contaminating all the results. So the test was dropped. But not to be put off, other tests were brought out, hailed as the *deus ex machina*, and the fact that obviously hypothyroid patients were still being missed, ignored. This is the problem with thyroid blood tests today. More later. We were going to talk about signs…

Very often the patient is overweight, a problem which may well cause very great distress. Not all patients are though; especially if there is a component of adrenal weakness, they may even be quite thin. A touch of the hand may reveal sometimes glacial coldness, in spite of wearing more jumpers and jackets than would seem appropriate. The face may be puffy with swelling and perhaps bags around the eyes. The voice may be hoarse, the speech slow. Scalp hair may be fine and thinning; one splendid textbook sign is the loss of some of the eyebrows, characteristically the outer third, together perhaps with loss of eyelashes. Skin coarse and puffy and the complexion is sallow; nails thin and flaking. One may be struck by some slowness of thought, a failure to grasp your meaning. They may sound generally low and depressed. The tongue may be revealing: often it looks over-large (and this may well be complained of) with shallow notches around the margins formed by the pressure of the teeth.

Blood pressure may be normal, raised or lowered; but what would be most often seen is a reduced pulse pressure. Let me explain this. You know that the blood pressure has a top and bottom component – say 130/70. With hypothyroidism, the top component becomes less and the bottom one more; in the above example it might become 120/80. In the over-active thyroid the reverse is the case, the pulse pressure widens and it might become 140/60, for example.

The pulse itself is characteristically slowed. If we consider the normal pulse to be, say, 72 beats per minute, the pulse may be down to 60. Again, in the over-active thyroid, the reverse is the case and the pulse may be 85 or 90. The hypothyroid pulse is not only slow but feels soft when it is taken at the wrist, whereas the hyperthyroid pulse is full and bounding.

On more general examination, the heart may be quite difficult to hear because it is running, as it were, below speed. Swelling of the ankles may be noticed. Reflexes are commonly slowed, most noticeably the Achilles reflex. This is the ankle reflex and if you want to try it at home; kneel on a chair and ask someone to sharply tap (with the edge of their hand, or a book) the big tendon above and behind the anklebone. The foot flicks up and then down to where it was. This return is what you are looking for. It should be instant and brisk. If the return is delayed or slow you have evidence for a slowed metabolism. It should be noted that this occurs with poor adrenal function as well.

With early hypothyroidism, the signs may not be all that striking, although the story should be pretty convincing. This is one reason why blood tests are turned to – especially if you haven't time to listen to the patient. But there is another simple sign, which will virtually without exception, put the matter beyond doubt. Originally reported in August 1942 in the *Journal of the American Medical Association* and later described in the *Lancet* in 1945 – and as true today as it was then – by Dr Broda Barnes, it has the merit of extreme simplicity, and anyone can do it for themselves. It is called the basal temperature test.

The Basal Temperature Test

Now, your body temperature is maintained remarkably very level, by various biological mechanisms, at 98.4°F, which is about 37°C. Like all mammals, this is what it means to be warm-blooded. Biological machinery and chemistry work better at these sorts of temperatures and indeed some mammals and birds are warmer than this. Reptiles cannot control their body temperature, and are sluggish when they are cold, becoming brisk when the sun has warmed them up. (If you think about it, 98.4°F is a pretty high temperature to run at; if the outside temperature reaches this level when we are on holiday for instance, we are not happy at all.) Fuel has to be burnt every moment of our lives to achieve this optimum temperature – which is why we need to eat three or four times a day. And why, if we don't eat, we get cold; our body temperature, at least on the outside, drops. Blood vessels close off and less heat is lost. Further heat loss becomes hypothermia and various essential mechanisms start to shut down until eventually the whole lot stops.

The rate of fuel burning is our metabolism, and it is the thyroid which controls this. You may remember that this control is exercised within the cell in the mitochondria, which are responsible for carbohydrate (sugars and starches – our body fuel) being combined with oxygen which we breathe in from the air, to provide energy, releasing carbon dioxide and water as waste products of this chemical reaction. So is maintained our body temperature. Since this is down to the thyroid hormone, you won't I am sure be surprised to learn that if this is low, then your temperature is likely to drop as well. Other factors help to hold it steady; muscular activity releases heat; putting on extra clothes prevents loss, as does a nice hot cup of tea. But if the temperature is taken under basal conditions, then the true picture is revealed. Basal means at total rest, as when you are asleep. Everybody's temperature drops when they are asleep, but not by very much: a few tenths of a degree only. But those with low thyroid function are not so fortunate; the body temperature drops as much as 3°F or 2°C. No wonder they feel tired and sluggish in the morning!

Now while it is not practical for us to take our temperature while asleep, it really is just as useful to take it *immediately on waking*. This is the basal temperature test, and how easy it is. Three minutes in the mouth on waking for an ordinary mercury glass thermometer, taking a bit less for an electric one; and just two or three seconds with an ear thermometer. Dr Barnes suggested ten minutes with a mercury thermometer in the armpit as being preferable, since a post nasal drip (very common in hypothyroidism) or a sore throat or sinusitis, could falsely elevate the oral temperature. Armpit temperatures are about ½ degree lower and some people seem to have very cold armpits. Nothing to stop you doing both though. The temperature *must* be done on waking – not after a cup of tea, or seeing to the baby, or going to the bathroom. Make sure the mercury thermometer is shaken down the *night before*; and if you are too bleary eyed to read it there and then, come back to it. You need to do it as many times – certainly no less than half a dozen – as you can, to average out the readings since they vary slightly and mysteriously from day to day. Clearly, you must be free of any other infection, like a cold or flu and so on, which would bring your temperature up.

For the ladies, things are a little different: if you are menstruating there are other hormonal factors at work, notably progesterone output, which affects the body temperature. It turns out that it is best to do the waking temperature on the second, third, fourth and fifth days of the cycle. Always write it all down so that you have visible evidence for yourself and your doctor.

This excellent and valuable home test is derided by many establishment doctors I am sorry to say. They are very wrong to do so and you must not listen to them. They will tell you that other things can lower body temperature and therefore it is not reliable. Well, there are some things you have to be sure about, so we will list them.[1]

1.   **Malnutrition.** This doesn't affect us in the UK particularly, unless we are in a real diet situation. So eat normally.

2.   **Alcoholism.** A really good drink dilates capillaries in the skin so you lose heat; if you were on the tiles the night before don't bother with the temperature, except to give yourself a fright.

3.   **Liver disease.** Certain liver diseases may cause low body temperature – but you'd have plenty of other problems and are unlikely to allow these to confuse you.

4.   **Hypothermia.** This can happen in the elderly with poorly heated homes.

You may well be told that many people run at these low temperatures naturally; and of course there are variations in the population. But many of these 'naturally' low people are actually hypothyroid, without knowing it.

So we can set limits to allow for normal variations. If your waking temperature is 97.6°F or 36.5°C or less, you may be hypothyroid and should consider carefully everything you have read so far. In all my years in the management of thyroid conditions, I have never known the basal temperature test to play me false if considered along with the symptoms and signs you have learnt about. Obviously the lower the readings are the more likely the diagnosis. The actual levels will give you some idea of how severe the thyroid deficiency actually is.

This most useful test will not only reveal early hypothyroidism, and put 'normal' blood tests properly in their place, but can be used to monitor your response to treatment, which of course we will soon come to. We should not expect dramatic changes overnight; it may take weeks or months for a fully established response to cause a temperature rise; nor will it, most likely, come back completely to normal, usually remaining obstinately a bit down. If your replacement dose is inadvertently high, however, an unexpected rise in the basal temperature will show that.

All my patients have been expected to do the basal temperature before initial consultation and use it in the subsequent monitoring of their treatment. Very useful as well is the pulse rate taken first thing with the temperature. Most people can find their own pulse, although the early morning hypothyroid pulse may be very soft and difficult to find. A simple device to measure the pulse (pulseometer) may be inexpensively obtained from most chemists. In any event you count the number of beats, best of all for 1 minute, or for ½ minute x 2, or if you are really busy 15 seconds x 4. Do remember to write it down. An unusually slow pulse is significant and as it speeds up it provides a most useful measure of your treatment. Since it rises quite soon (quicker than the temperature) it helps you gauge your treatment response.

You are now able to make your own diagnosis. You will be told it's not thyroid dysfunction, but depression, anxiety, hypochondria, or nothing at all. Have the courage of your convictions. You have nothing to lose but your chains.

Blood Tests

As you may have gathered by now, I deeply deplore the tendency in modern medicine to diagnose by machine, or computer printout, relegating the doctor to a pusher of buttons, and reader of bits of paper. The slow decline in medical standards, and particularly, the relationship between doctors and patients is in part due to this. In no medical condition has this been more damaging than in the diagnosis and treatment of hypothyroidism. Thousands of people in the United Kingdom, Europe, Australia, New Zealand and the USA, suffer a variable degree of ill-health which is unnecessary and ruins the lives of patients and their families. Anxiety in the medical establishment about rules and dogma has led to a slavish reliance on blood tests, which are often unreliable and can actually produce a false picture of the true situation. I have seen patients who have had several successive blood tests because the doctor very properly suspected a thyroid problem but could find no abnormality until perhaps the fourth or fifth test, by which time the patient had had worsening symptoms for further months or years. Only then, and all too late, does the doctor feel justified in treating the patient whose life has by now been irrevocably changed by depression, chronic ill-health, perhaps loss of job and destruction of home relationships. I have seen patients whose hypothyroidism is so severe that they actually have myxoedema, but they are treated for fluid retention with diuretics; for depression and exhaustion with antidepressants, for constipation with opening medicine, and for excess weight by rigorous dieting. And all the time the diagnosis could have been made by just looking at the patient.

So it is time we looked at the blood tests, so often regarded as a matter of faith and heresy to question. As I have said, there have been quite a number of different tests in years gone by; these that follow are in use today.

Thyroid Stimulating Hormone (TSH)

Regarded as sensitive and impossible to be wrong is the test for TSH. The level of this rises in the bloodstream as the thyroid starts to fail; the pituitary gland attempts to flog the thyroid into producing more thyroid hormone by increasing the level of TSH it makes under the control of the hypothalamus. Normal levels are quoted as around 0.15 micro units per millilitre (μU/ml) as the lower level, and anything from 3.5 to 6.0 μU/ml as the upper limit, depending on the laboratory. These figures are crucial, since if you are within this range you will be told you are normal – *whatever the symptoms.* Almost as bad is to be told 'you are borderline' and 'come back in six months'. As a result of this test, thousands are denied treatment. The American Association of Clinical Endocrinologists quote 0.3 to 3.0 μU/ml as the optimal range to aim for. In fact, a level of 2 μU/ml should arouse suspicion, and anything over 2.5 should be diagnostic.[2, 3] Given the view from the US, it is hard to understand why very recently in the United Kingdom, a level of over 10 μU/ml has been suggested as being necessary before treatment is offered.

Thyroxine (T4)

The thyroid hormone, thyroxine (T4) is also commonly measured. This is transported around the bloodstream attached to a protein fraction, although some T4 is free of this attachment. So the test measures 'Total' thyroxine and 'Free' thyroxine. Normal levels, which vary from laboratory to laboratory, are around 60 – 155 nanomols per litre (nmol/l). Free thyroxine is much less: normal levels are around 9 – 28 picomols per litre (pmols/l).

Tri-iodothyronine (T3)

Also is measured the active thyroid hormone tri-iodothyronine (T3), which has been converted from T4. Some of this too is attached to a protein transporter; so is measured Total T3, 1.1 – 2.6 nmol/l and Free T3, 3 – 8 pmols/l.

Thyroid Antibodies

Finally, is measured the thyroid antibody fraction as thyroperoxidase (TPO) and thyroglobulin (TgAb) which will certainly indicate thyroid damage as in Hashimoto's disease and any other autoimmune thyroiditis.

Why blood tests can be unreliable

Sadly, I have to say that all these measurements (except the last) may be so flawed that treatment based on them is bound to be wrong. So what goes wrong? And why are doctors not aware that they may be so badly off beam?

We now need to examine the reasons blood tests may be so flawed. First and foremost these are only measures of the levels of thyroid hormone in the *blood*. What we need to know is the level of thyroid in the tissues, and, of course, this the blood test cannot tell us. The nearest we can go is the basal temperature test, or the basal metabolic rate; the first we have discussed; the second is now of historical value. The patient was connected up to a device that measured oxygen uptake and carbon dioxide excretion; the rate of usage determined the metabolic rate; this is also subject to various errors.

The amount of thyroid hormones being carried by the bloodstream varies in a highly dynamic way, and may be up at one point and down the next. The blood test is simply a two-dimensional snapshot of the situation *at that moment*. The slowed circulation may cause haemo-concentration from fluid loss, so that the apparent thyroid levels are higher than they should be. (A simple way to explain this is to think of a spoonful of sugar in your cup of tea. If it is only half a cup of tea but you still put in your teaspoon of sugar, then although the amount of sugar is the same, the tea will be twice as sweet.)

The blood levels depend mostly on what's happening to the thyroid hormones. If the cellular receptors are sluggish, or resistant, or there is extra tissue fluid, together with mucopolysaccharides, the thyroid won't enter the cells as it should; so that part of the hormone is unused and left behind, giving a falsely higher reading to the blood test. It is simply building up unused hormone. This may apply to both T3 and T4. Further complications exist if the T4 → T3 conversion is not working properly, with a 5'-deiodinase enzyme deficiency. There will be too much T4, and too little T3. If there is a conversion block, *and* a T3 receptor uptake deficiency, both T3 and T4 may be normal or even raised. The patient will be diagnosed as normal or even over-active, in spite of all other evidence to the contrary. It grieves me to report that I have intervened several times to prevent patients, diagnosed as hyperthyroid, having an *under-active* thyroid removed when the only evidence was the high T4 level (due to receptor resistance) and the patient was clinically obviously hypothyroid.

Adrenal insufficiency adds another dimension for error to the T4 and T3 tests. Adrenal insufficiency, of which more anon, will adversely affect thyroid production, conversion, tissue uptake and thyroid response. It may make a complete nonsense of the blood tests.

The most commonly used test of all is the TSH. I have sadly come across very few doctors who can accept the fact that a normal, or low TSH, may still occur with a low thyroid. The doctrine is high TSH = low thyroid. Normal TSH = normal thyroid. But the pituitary may not be working properly (secondary or tertiary hypothyroidism). It may not be responding to the thyrotrophin release hormone (TRH) produced by the hypothalamus, which itself may not be producing enough TRH for reasons we saw earlier. The pituitary may be damaged by the low thyroid state anyway, and be sluggish in its TSH output.

Thyroid workers like Dr John Lowe, the Barnes Foundation, Thierry and Theresa Hertoghe in Belgium, and me too, have been aware that blood tests may not just be useless, but worse than useless, since sick people are sent packing, or are given the wrong treatment. Doctors hence are obliged by an unbending establishment to do these tests, whether they believe them or not, or be accused of malpractice. In the USA all doctors working under the auspices of the Barnes Foundation do these tests on every patient – but then go on to treat their patients clinically, irrespective of what the tests say. This, of course, is my argument. As doctors, use your common sense, and enter a partnership with your patient. Your patient will tell you how they are feeling a damn sight better than any blood test.

While it is perfectly proper to make a clinical diagnosis of a thyroid dysfunction, and treat the complaint, there *is* a place for blood tests, and where practical, I would usually undertake them. It is useful to do other blood tests such as a full blood count, chemistry, liver function tests, and perhaps hormone tests. The problem is usually a practical one. The NHS doctor has his budget to think of; and in the private sector the tests I have mentioned could easily cost £150. For accurate and inexpensive thyroid and other hormone tests, available to all, you may contact private laboratories (contact details found in Appendix D).

One final word. During the last few years alternatives to the blood tests have been made available. One is the 24 hour urine test, where a sample of urine collected over 24 hours is measured for T4 and T3. This test shows the T3 and T4 which has been used in 24 hours, rather than what is present in the bloodstream, where a proportion may not have been properly used as I explained. This is therefore a good deal more sensitive than the standard tests, although convincing doctors may be another matter.[4] The Red Apple Clinic and IWDL (via Thyroid UK) do this test in the United Kingdom. DiagnosTech, an American company, undertake a salivary test for thyroid, a relatively new technique not yet fully validated.

Other Thyroid Problems

Most distressing can be marked enlargement of the thyroid, which may be symmetrical or asymmetrical. This, the goitre, we mentioned above, may be due to a number of factors. We saw earlier that iodine deficiency will cause chronic enlargement; but this is rarely seen today except in remote inland areas. Many people develop a diffuse, usually soft enlargement, especially teenage girls, with no real symptoms requiring attention. Sometimes these quietly disappear, but they may progress to become rather harder and with lumps and nodules over the years. It is then called multi-nodular goitre, and may be inconvenient or unsightly. At this point medical advice should be sought. X-rays and ultrasound may show its full extent, and whether further tests or intervention are required. One such is the use of a radioactive isotope of iodine (I_{131}), which is taken up to a greater degree by the abnormally active thyroid nodules and will show up as hot spots on a thyroid scan, providing a picture of the thyroid tissue health.

It is more common for the thyroid to present a nodule as a lump one side or the other. Many of these patients will have the tests mentioned above, but most often will have the nodule drained by a fine needle. (Fine needle aspiration (FNA) for the technically minded.) The fluid and cells are subjected to microscopy. At this point cancer cells may be looked for, which is why a growing nodule is not something you should try to deal with yourself. Fortunately, cancer is really quite rare and has a very high survival rate (95% overall); the average practice may not see more than one case every few years or so.

For the sake of completeness I am going briefly to list the types of thyroid cancer that occur. Early on in life, and in young women, the cancer is likely to be papillary cancer (from its frond like appearance under the microscope). Later on in life, after about the age of 30, the cancer is more likely to be follicular cancer. Much rarer are medullary, lymphoma, or anaplastic cancer, the last two really only occurring in older age groups. Treatment is essentially surgical; the whole gland is removed, together with any associated glands with papillary cancer; some tissue may safely be left in surgical treatment of the follicular form. Any stray cancer cells are mopped up by a course of radioactive iodine a few weeks after the surgery and before thyroid replacement has been started. It is considered good practice to prevent thyroid stimulation, as by the TSH, to prevent recurrence; so thyroid replacement ensures the TSH is kept very low.

Thyroid eye disease (TED) may be a complication of thyroid dysfunction one would rather have done without. The first thing to say is that it affects, in at least 90% of cases, people with an over-active thyroid (Graves' disease). Rarely it may be seen in Hashimoto's disease.

The fatty tissue behind the eyes swells for reasons which are really not clear, but may be part of the autoimmune reaction which initially causes the thyroid over-activity. The presence of an immunoglobulin which competes with TSH at the TSH receptor sites has been suggested by some workers,[5] and been called long acting thyroid stimulator (LATS). The target receptors are identified as TSHR-ab and seem to be particularly involved in the processes of thyroid eye disease, causing the exophthalmos. This has the main effect of pushing the eye forward to some extent and this becomes noticeable when the patient develops a stare, with the eyes beginning to bulge. The patient becomes aware of gritty or sore eyes and there may be discomfort moving the eyes. Double vision may also occur, and puffiness around the eyes may prove difficult to treat.

The condition may not occur at the same time as the thyroid over-activity, but develops later. It doesn't seem that successful treatment of the thyroid condition necessarily improves the eye problems. Radioactive iodine treatment of the over-active thyroid has come under some suspicion; most physicians are concerned that this treatment of Graves' disease doesn't help thyroid eye disease, or may even make it worse. Steroid supplementation in the initial stages of this treatment may be helpful, and recent work has shown that quite high doses have been very effective.

The condition usually settles after a while, although surgical intervention has been found necessary sometimes. It seems that smoking has a generally negative effect though. Treatment is usually to use lubricant (hypromellose) eye drops. If things are worsening, ophthalmologist advice should be sought. Help with altered vision and the use of immune suppressive treatment (usually corticosteroids) may be given. Sometimes surgery is suggested and counselling may be offered for the facial changes due to excessively protuberant eyes. The organisation to help and provide advice is the Thyroid Eye Disease Association (TED), a self-help group (see Appendix D).

Although you may be becoming anxious about getting on with the treatment, there is a major additional problem we need to look at in more depth first. This is the adrenal connection.

Chapter Seven

Iodine, Other Hormones and the Thyroid

Part A – The Role of Iodine

As we saw earlier, iodine is very important to thyroid function. You will have learnt that a shortage of dietary iodine will cause goitre and hypothyroidism. In England we call this Derbyshire Neck, the result of very little iodine in the soil. Fish contain a lot of iodine, so in coastal areas deficiencies do not occur. It might be thought to be a simple cause and effect. But, alas, it is not as simple as that.

Iodine actually has a number of parts to play:

1. It is essential for the production of the thyroid hormone, detailed below.

2. Iodine is a trigger for a process called apoptosis, or programmed cell death. This is where the cells in our bodies die as part of a useful ongoing process. (Skin cells have to die and be lost on a continuous basis, for example.)

3. Iodine, together with the thyroid hormones, has a monitoring and surveillance role, finding and destroying abnormal cells (like pre-cancer cells). Iodine also has an antioxidant and an anti-free radical action.

4. Proteins with allergenic potential may get wrapped and coated with iodine, thus rendering them inactive.

5. Iodine has a protective and preventative effect against *Helicobacter pylori*, the bacterium that lives in the stomach and causes ulcers and stomach cancer.

6. The tissues of the breast have a particular affinity for iodine (notably in pregnancy and lactation) and desensitise breast glandular tissue to the activity of oestrogen.

7. Iodine is a powerful antiseptic and may be used topically in complete safety, working even in high dilutions.

Iodine was first discovered in seaweed just after the beginning of the 19th century, and a French chemist, Gay-Lussac, gave it its name. It was also found that the ash of burnt seaweed shrank goitres, and later, by Dr Marine and Dr Larsen working in America, that iodine deficiency was associated with goitres in all mammals. So let's have a look at why iodine is important to the thyroid.

The thyroid hormone manufacturing cells in the thyroid gland are called follicular cells, and they contain a protein material called colloid. The colloid cells of the thyroid take up iodide ions from various iodine compounds in our diet and convert them to elemental iodine. This now combines with the amino acid tyrosine and the chain of building through T1, T2, T3 to T4 (thyroxine) now occurs. Amino acids are the building blocks of protein and we use some 22 of them in various combinations. You will recall that tyrosine made up into two tyrosyl rings and one iodine atom forms the thyroid hormone mono-iodothyronine (T1); with two iodine atoms it is called di-iodothyronine (T2). With an extra iodine atom we have formed tri-iodothyronine (T3), and then tetra-iodothyronine (T4) with, of course, four iodine atoms.

A deficiency of iodine intake increases the secretion of TSH from the pituitary, and lessens the manufacture of T4. The balance of T3 to the amount of T4 is disturbed, and the amount of T3 becomes relatively more in proportion to T4, even though both are reduced.

Taking in *an excess* of iodide has quite a different effect. The iodine now causes the biosynthetic enzymes in the thyroid to *reduce* their activity, with the effect of reducing thyroid output, though the TSH may be raised. Goitre formation may be induced and thus eventually hypothyroidism. Marine showed that 2 grams of potassium iodide twice a year was sufficient to prevent hypothyroidism due to low ingestion of iodine, and more recently, Larson in 1974 showed that patients on abnormal diets restricted in iodine salts, or on diuretics for an extended time, so reduced the iodine pool that hypothyroidism could result. Worth noting too is that pregnant women require extra iodine, but not too much or the baby may be rendered hypothyroid. Adult needs are thought to be no more than about 100–200 mcg daily. It might be of further interest to note that in coastal regions of Japan where they eat a great deal of fish, the high levels of iodine raise the incidence of hypothyroidism to 2 or 3 times the average.

The aspect of thyroid hormone and iodine that is extremely important to us is the effect on breast tissue. Broda Barnes showed four decades ago[1] that if the thyroid status was normal, with thyroid supplementation if required, then his patients simply didn't get breast cancer. Other workers, Venturi, Eskin, and Derry, showed that iodine had a similar effect; the iodine prevented the cystic hyperplasia (lumpy breast tissue), which may be a precursor to breast cancer.[2, 3, 4] It may be that a high iodine intake largely prevents breast cancer, although the fatty acid derivative EPA in the fish may be playing a role. Japanese women, who, as we saw, eat a lot of fish and therefore iodine rarely get breast cancer; this was also true of Icelandic ladies, but they now enjoy a more European diet, and notably suffer increasingly from breast cancer.[5] Most of these ladies had small thyroids due to the abundance of dietary iodine and now many of them have developed hypothyroidism.

Careful research has shown that excess iodine may shut down the thyroid in people with marginal thyroid function; indeed, it can be used for a short period to reduce the activity of the over-active thyroid. This places us in something of a quandary. Iodine has a number of beneficial effects in the body as a whole, and protects against breast cancer. Dr Derry, in Canada, believes that 2-3 mg of Lugol's Iodine daily will prevent breast cancer, though the recommended standard daily dose is much less than this (100–200 mcg daily). Clearly then, this higher dose of iodine may lower thyroid activity; and if a substantial dose of iodine is to be used, the thyroid activity must be carefully monitored.

It is clear that patients with pre-existing thyroid disease (notably Hashimoto's disease by ironic coincidence) are abnormally sensitive to excess iodine, and even a small excess may cause a small but significant reduction in thyroid output.

To summarise, iodine may first of all render blood tests unreliable. Too little has been proven to cause goitre and hypothyroidism, but a well meant surplus intake may well have the reverse effect to that intended, and cause yet again goitre and hypothyroidism.

The moral of the story. Most women do need extra iodine, but the amount is difficult to specify. Too much may well cause hypothyroidism, so this needs careful thought and the danger signals of low thyroid must be watched for.

Part B – Oestrogen, Progesterone & Testosterone

The hormones that keep us male and female are crucially affected by thyroid and adrenal function, and in turn can affect the proper functioning of the thyroid itself. So let us see where they fit in.

Since my approach to metabolic problems is holistic, we have to ask if thyroid and adrenal insufficiency may be altered or worsened by deficiencies elsewhere. The answer is, of course, yes. Since a state of lowered metabolism means that nothing really works as it was designed to, it follows that other hormone producing glands may not do their job properly either. It is a bit like an extraordinarily complex piece of electrical machinery, designed for 240 volts, running on 210 volts. It runs, but the lights look dim and flicker a bit. Bringing up the voltage – gently – will get everything working again.

So far as other components of the endocrine system go, we must be prepared for partial recovery only, and supplementation may well be indicated elsewhere as well. We are talking mostly about sex hormones here, and the effects of the menopause on both sexes. We have learnt already how important the adrenal corticosteroids are in the maintenance of the body's normal health; the male and female sex hormones, which are of course also steroids, are just as extraordinarily important in their own right. (It may have perhaps surprised you to realise that the whole body, most especially many of its hormones, is based on the steroid molecule. The use of the word 'steroid' has been denigrated in the popular mind as being potentially, if not actually, dangerous, and this is a complete distortion. The contraceptive pill, for which millions of prescriptions are written weekly, is based on two steroids and few doctors or patients are especially concerned that they do in fact belong to the great family of steroids.)

So we need to have a look at the whole business, to enable us to decide to intervene if necessary while treating the metabolic problems. Women actually produce three different sex hormones, oestrogen (which has three different forms: oestradiol, oestrone and oestriol), progesterone and testosterone. You thought testosterone was a male hormone, didn't you? Well, it is; but women produce it too – though less than men of course. (The reverse is also the case.) Oestradiol, the main oestrogen, mostly comes from the ovaries, but all three are produced by the adrenal glands, directly or indirectly, and more so after the menopause.

The way it all works is this. As the **menarche** (the start of periods) approaches, the ovaries start to produce oestrogen and under the influence of a pituitary hormone, the follicle stimulating hormone (FSH), an ovarian follicle (of which there are many hundreds, each containing an egg cell waiting its time) matures an ovum, which surfaces about mid-cycle and is released. It finds its way into one of the fallopian tubes (right or left, depending on which ovary produced the ovum) where it may or may not be fertilised. The place from where it was released on the ovary undergoes a change to produce the corpus luteum or 'yellow body'. This structure begins to produce, under the influence of luteinising hormone (LH) from the pituitary, another hormone, progesterone. This prepares the lining of the womb for implantation if the ovum is fertilised. Oestrogen and progesterone are produced together for the second half of the cycle; and then the supply is cut off abruptly, which starts off the menstrual period. Figure 9 below shows this cycle.

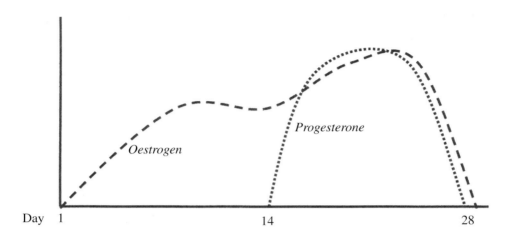

Day 1   14   28

Figure 9. Oestrogen and progesterone levels through the menstrual cycle

Hypothyroidism can affect this process in several ways. To start with, a low thyroid state affects the onset of the first period. The first period may come unusually early at 8, 9 or 10 years old; or, it may come unusually late, at 15, 16 or 17 years old. Periods starting abnormally like this should raise a suspicion about the thyroid at once.

The periods may be abnormal in other ways. They may be exceedingly painful with collapse and prostration of the unfortunate girl; they may be very heavy or very light or come at irregular times. There may be premenstrual tension to make life miserable. These problems may occur at any time of life, but may sort themselves out a bit after having children.

In the later thirties and early forties there is the **premenopause** state, when the oestrogen/progesterone levels start to fall and it all starts to go wrong. Flooding and terrible premenstrual tension (PMT) (or, as the Americans call it, PMS or premenstrual syndrome) may ruin things so badly that relationships suffer.[6] Some doctors won't have it that PMT occurs at all. I remember reading an authoritative article by a lady doctor who discounted it completely; one just wonders what planet she came from. It seems to me not only is it a very real problem; if anything, it is getting worse. Although a number of causes have been cited, it seems clear that it is associated with an imbalance between the oestrogen and progesterone production.

It is at this point, of course, that hysterectomy becomes the treatment of choice, and worn out with it all, the unhappy sufferer consents to surgery. Relief from the terrible periods may well justify the hysterectomy for the patient; but this approach may have missed the point altogether. As I said earlier, hysterectomy is very likely to affect thyroid activity. There seems to be a chemical dialogue between the womb and the thyroid, and in my experience, interference such as sterilisation, termination, or even a D&C (dilation and curretage), seems to damage thyroid function for many.

The weight gain that nearly always occurs after hysterectomy is almost certainly not due to comfort eating while grieving for one's lost fertility, but because thyroid activity may have been further damaged. This, and the other symptoms of a decline in thyroid activity, is a heavy price to pay for an operation which may well not have been necessary and could have been avoided if thyroid status had been properly assessed and treated.

Throughout my experience with low thyroid, I have been staggered to find that some women lose their PMT within a month or so of starting their thyroid supplementation – simply the result of improved progesterone production. Where progesterone production in the mid thirties and forties has not been improved by thyroid supplementation, and as oestrogen dominance brings with it its own problems of bloating, weight gain, mood swings and increased risk of cancer, thought must be given to progesterone supplementation.

Following the premenopause state is the **perimenopause**, where commonly progesterone starts to fail first; which allows the oestrogen dominant situation to really take over and causes worsening of pre-menstrual tension, breast enlargement and weight gain. Again the poor sufferer may feel hysterectomy is her only option. The problem with relatively high oestrogen levels is that they reduce thyroid hormone production and the tissue uptake, which is why, when the menopause is in full swing, you get extra fatigue and weight gain. This all finally shades into the **menopausal** state, where eventually, the oestrogen starts to fail as well. For some women it is an abrupt thing, there one month and gone the next. Very often the process is rather more protracted than this; the periods start lengthening and sputter about; they may become heavy with pain and flooding, or become very light and irregular. It causes mood changes, poor skin and hair condition, excess facial hair, osteoporosis, atrophic vaginitis and loss of libido. All this will be hastened or worsened by a low thyroid/adrenal state.

Hormone replacement therapy (HRT) will usually consist of both oestrogen and progesterone, preferably in a cream form. The standard way of doing this is by the use of a group of artificial progesterones, which are called progestogens and the synthetic hormone Norithesterone is an example. While these may well be helpful for some women, they have a number of side effects which have made them less and less popular and an alternative must be sought. Of increasing popularity nowadays is the use of natural progesterone, which is actually extracted from plants. It is incorporated in creams which may be simply rubbed into the skin daily: absorption through the skin turns out to be a very satisfactory form of supplementation. Although establishment thinking is, as might be expected, somewhat suspicious of the natural product, favouring the artificial, very many thousands of women are greatly benefiting from transdermal progesterone (see Appendix D).

The effect of the menopause in men is obviously similar. The older man in the normal way suffers a loss of testosterone with age, which is variable in degree and rate of loss. The **male menopause**, however, is a very real thing, which of course men are often not prepared to admit to. It will cause general tiredness, loss of drive and vigour, loss of potency, coarsening of the skin, hair loss over the body as a whole, loss of upright posture and osteoporosis. The difference between the male menopause (which we now call the 'andropause') and the female menopause, is that it is likely to be on a longer time scale and not marked by any specific event. The important thing to recognise is that it is hastened and worsened by loss of thyroid function, and one may well find that one is dealing with low thyroid, low adrenal reserve and low testosterone as all part of the hypothyroid state. While providing support for the low thyroid output is likely to improve testosterone output to a degree, it is only common sense to check testosterone levels and provide adequate support in this direction as well.

This may be carried out in two ways. Testosterone undecanoate, marketed as Restandol, may be given in any dose from 1 to 6 capsules daily, depending on need. Its expense makes it an unpopular prescription from NHS doctors, although a private prescription may be more willingly given. The use of an intramuscular injection monthly, of Sustanon 250 (which consists of four kinds of testosterone salts to provide gradual release into the system over the month) is very much cheaper; my view is that it works better than the oral form. Best of all though is a transdermal cream. Its effectiveness may be monitored by a blood test, which may be relied upon. It is good practice to have a check done (usually at the initial blood test) of the prostatic specific antigen (PSA), which is a marker or early warning of prostatic cancer. Further research to improve the reliability of this test is underway at present, which is of considerable importance since prostatic cancer appears to be on the increase.[7] If cancer is present, testosterone will not be given, since it 'feeds' the growth; although conversely, if there is no sign of a problem the evidence is that testosterone protects against cancer.

One last thought. There is a most alarming gap in the management of infertility and this is the failure to realise that a prime and gravely neglected cause is hypothyroidism. It is obvious that there are several ways the healthy ovum can be affected: its production, its maturation, proper fertilisation and implantation. The male of the species is affected too: spermatozoa are more likely to be diminished in numbers and less fertile – apart from the fact that a loss of libido affects men and women equally. I pointed out earlier that women produce testosterone, though less than men, of course. Women need testosterone for health and well-being and it is what mostly drives the female libido. For both sexes testosterone in addition acts as a natural anabolic steroid; that is, as a hormone which encourages the creation of new tissues within the body, most particularly muscles and bones. The continued running down of testosterone is part of the ageing process for both men and women.

Part C – Pregnenolone, DHEA and Melatonin

Pregnenolone

Most people have somewhat vague ideas about the place of pregnenolone in the world of hormones, so I thought it was about time for a few words of explanation: about how it is made, what it does and how it relates to thyroid and adrenal problems.

Pregnenolone is made mostly in the adrenal glands, but small amounts are also made in the liver, sex glands, the brain and even the retina of the eye. About 14 mg daily is produced on average, but this declines with age. It has been known about since 1940 but only in the last two decades or so has attention been drawn to it as advances in the understanding of how hormones work have been made.

The first thing we must do is to establish what pregnenolone actually is and what it is made of. You may be surprised to learn that the precursor of pregnenolone is actually our old friend cholesterol. Cholesterol is actually a much maligned substance; it is essential as the basis of much of our hormone chemistry, and, something I mentioned earlier, the body actually makes 80% of all the cholesterol in our system. Anyway, cholesterol is converted to pregnenolone, which becomes the, as it were, grandmother of the adrenal hormones. (It might help if you glanced at the flow chart at the end of this section.) From it, three groups of hormones are synthesised within, principally, the adrenals.

As you will see, the first pathway is the mineralocorticoids, the second, the glucocorticoids and the third, the androgens. Many of the processes link up and some can go into reverse. The end result of the first pathway is to provide a mechanism for regulating the fluid balance and sodium and potassium levels in the bloodstream via aldosterone. The second group finishes up with the production of cortisol, which helps the system face chronic stress and helps to regulate sugar balance in the bloodstream. The third pathway finishes up with DHEA (dehydroepiandrosterone), which may be turned, as the body requires, into testosterone and/or oestrogen. DHEA has a story of its own and I shall cover this next; it is widely used in the system and has a number of important benefits.

The suspicion was that pregnenolone might well have various direct effects apart from the vital hormones it turns into. It has to be said that there remain some gaps in the knowledge of all the roles it has to play, but one thing has emerged very forcefully: it is very safe and seems to have no long- or short-term undesirable side effects. (We are looking down a perspective of more than 40 years, and so can be pretty confident.)

The Nervous System

Animal studies[8] have shown clear evidence that pregnenolone enhances memory and learning. Since both brain and spinal cord can produce it, we must not be surprised that it activates receptors concerned with the stimulation of the brain. So pregnenolone is a neural hormone with cognitive enhancement properties.

Depressive Illness

The same neuro-endocrine response affects mood and behaviour response in the nervous system; in particular, low pregnenolone is associated with depressive illness. It has also proved very helpful in stress and many authorities believe it has a role to play in its management. It has been noticed that when one is under stress pregnenolone production increases.

Arthritis

Pregnenolone was originally used some 60 years ago, in the treatment of arthritis, with some considerable benefit. Its use, and research into it, was abruptly discontinued in the early 1950s when cortisone came to the fore. The effect of cortisone was more dramatic, and since cortisones could be synthesised and patented – pregnenolone cannot be patented – cortisone took over. Sadly, as we know, the side effects of overused synthetic cortisone then became apparent and nowadays the use of cortisone is very much more carefully monitored.

Skin

Back in 1962 some workers[9] used pregnenolone (in the form of a cream) on elderly ladies with wrinkles, and the good news was that there was notable benefit.

The bad news was that the wrinkles came back after it was stopped. The authors considered that the effect was probably due to hydration, and no-one else has looked into the question. Pregnenolone is made commercially from a substance, extracted from wild yams in Mexico, called diosgenin (as is the natural progesterone cream). One company that provides an excellent preparation is Pharmwest (see Appendix D). A dose of 30 mg daily is usually thought to be about right.

Figure 10. Adrenal Hormone Flow Chart

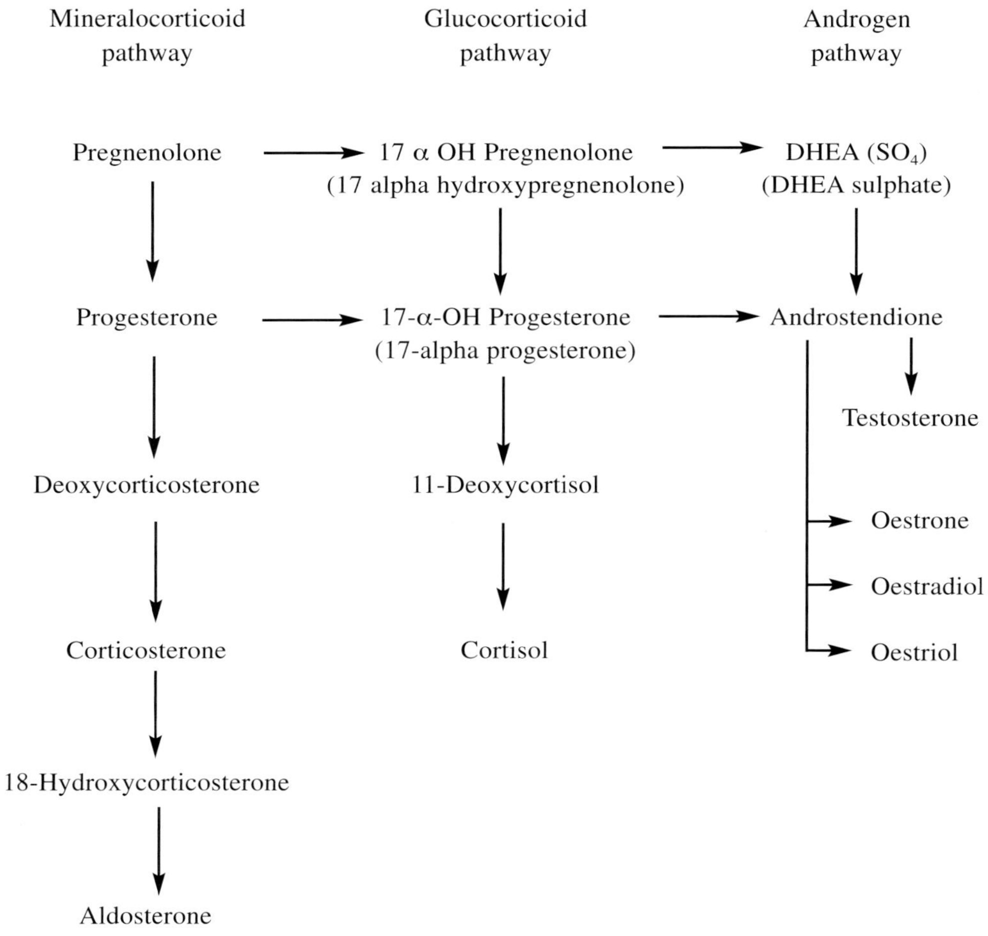

DHEA

There is one more hormone which may be affected by a low metabolic state, and that is DHEA, which we remember comes from the adrenal glands. It stands for Dehydroepiandrosterone, and is one of the many steroid hormones on which our health and vitality depend. Very few people in the United Kingdom are likely to have heard of DHEA (although it is widely used in the USA) and its importance is poorly known among most doctors. Yet it is likely to become as familiar as, for example, HRT during the next decades, because it is turning out to be an integral part of our body's resistance to the diseases of ageing.

DHEA is made chiefly at two sites in the body. One, by our sex glands, the ovaries and testes. Two, when these decline with age, its manufacture switches to the outer part – the cortex – of our adrenal glands. It seems that the obvious role of DHEA is to act as a precursor to the sex hormones; but only a tenth of the total output is used for this purpose. The remainder has other purposes to accomplish in our systems and it is these we shall look at.

The chemical pathway of DHEA manufacture is worth understanding and a glance at the flowchart on page 101 will make this clear. It is the DHEA sulphate that does all the work, but the discussion is simplified if we drop the 'sulphate'. You will notice that DHEA can be turned into either testosterone or oestrogen and that to have a normal sex hormone level you need enough DHEA to start with.

Consequently, by supplementing DHEA it is likely that women will have extra oestrogen (restoring levels to normal), and men extra testosterone; it is tempting to suggest that whatever is low will be improved. (Remember that men have oestrogen, but less than women, and women have testosterone, but less than men.) Although in general men do not need extra oestrogen, women can benefit from testosterone in two ways: one, because of its useful effect on the circulation and anabolism (tissue building), and two, because it has a powerful role to play in the maintenance of the libido. One interesting thing to start with: the amount of DHEA made in the body is directly related to age; the older you are, the less you have. Cause and effect? We don't know for definite, although most authorities working in this field think so; but of course the sex hormone levels (of which DHEA is a precursor) also decline with age. Symptoms of DHEA deficiency include fatigue, loss of muscle tone, tremor and lack of well-being; it may be associated with autoimmune disease.

Research continues on the actual biological role of DHEA. First obesity. Several studies[10] have shown that weight loss occurs with DHEA, basically because it improves the calorie burning levels in our so-called 'brown fat'. (Brown fat is where the body gets rid of surplus calories, turning them into heat.) Possibly a related effect seems to be an anti-atherogenic effect; the ageing of arteries by arteriosclerosis is halted. Death rates, at least in men, from coronary heart disease, have been found to be reduced. Noticeable too is a reduction in excess cholesterol, and low-density lipoproteins, which are the 'nasty' triglycerides linked to cardiovascular disease.

The positive effects of DHEA are to block immune suppression, and balance the catabolic (tissue breakdown) effects of cortisone with its anabolic (tissue building) effects. It lowers cholesterol and glucose levels in the blood and has therefore the effect of reducing obesity. It has an important role to play in the maintenance of bone density, and additionally maintains the system's integrity by attacking free radicals. At least as interesting is a reducing effect on carcinogenesis, most notably breast cancer. Growth of tumour is definitely reduced. The inhibition of an enzyme which is increased in cancer, glucose-6-phosphate-dehydrogenase, is well documented.[11] Other studies[12, 13] showed that women with low DHEA were more likely to contract breast cancer than those where it was normal. Most important, DHEA is needed at cellular level to ensure normal receptor uptake of thyroid hormone.

Other workers[14] have targeted the central nervous system and found that DHEA acted as a neural facilitator; that is, memory and thinking were improved where DHEA was previously low. There was also a study showing a slowing in the ravages of Alzheimer's disease; survival of neurones was significantly improved. Discernible improvement was also found in multiple sclerosis sufferers, and another study showed improvement in chronic fatigue syndrome. Although these are early studies, they were statistically significant in their finding and should be taken seriously. Further studies are continuing.

Animal studies[15] have shown an improvement in immune response, when DHEA was added to their diets. Not only did the mice fight infection better, but they were more likely to overcome illness in general, including cancer. Another interesting effect was found in reducing the need for treatment of diabetes. Workers in Holland found that DHEA may protect against certain viral infections, including a modest inhibitory effect on HIV-1 (the Aids virus). Of great interest in this study, was that people with high DHEA levels didn't contract the syndrome as readily as those with low levels.[16]

To summarise, DHEA has a so far not well-understood role to play in the health and vitality of the body as a whole. But the evidence that it has a great deal to do with the diseases of ageing, arteriosclerosis and cardiovascular disease (including hypertension), and also obesity, immune response, AIDS, multiple allergies, diabetes and cancer, is overwhelming and will continue to accumulate. I consider that checking the DHEA is an important part of the screening program, and its replacement unhesitatingly part of the treatment of the ageing process. It is a natural substance and no significant side effects have ever been found in its use, even at relatively high doses, although an increase in hair growth and/or acne has occasionally been reported. This may be avoided by using a DHEA derivative called 7-keto DHEA, which has no androgenic potential.

I am certain that in time, replacement of DHEA will be as important as replacement of sex hormone (HRT) for both sexes.

Figure 11. DHEA flow chart

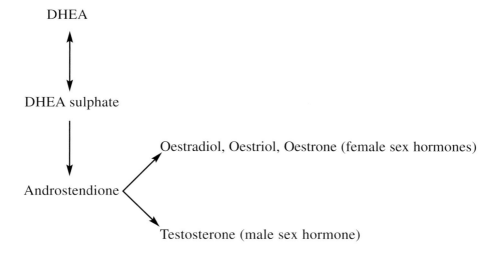

Melatonin

Until recently, the hormone melatonin had only a passing mention in most textbooks, and most people had never heard of it; it didn't seem actually to do anything much and had no medical applications. But with recent research and the now easy access to melatonin via the internet, it is time that both doctors and the public knew a lot more about it.

Before going into what it is, and what it does, let's see where it comes from. Well, as I explained earlier, it is made in the pineal gland, a pea-sized member of the family of endocrine glands. It is situated deep within the brain of the higher animals, covered by the cerebral cortex, but in lower animals it is so close to the top of the skull that it can detect light. It responds to the ambient light; the production of melatonin is controlled by the amount of light received by our eyes, so that the less light there is the more is made; bright sunlight shuts it off completely.

So what is melatonin for? Well, it has been known for some time that its most obvious role is in regulating our daily life rhythms – called circadian rhythms. The chief of these, of course, is sleep. As the shadows fall with the end of the day, melatonin is produced and is swept around the body by the bloodstream, slowing down biological activity in our tissues and shutting down the hormone outputs of other glands. So we are prepared for sleep. And as our systems run themselves down, we fall asleep. Breathing slows, our pulse rate slows, our blood pressure drops.

As we have seen, melatonin also controls much longer body rhythms: those of the seasons. In animals the changes needed to prepare for mating at special times of the year, for hibernation and for migration, are overseen by the pineal. Human beings with the artificial rhythms of civilization are less influenced in this way, but the control is still there; the seasonal variations in the birth rate are an echo of our evolutionary heritage with the pineal in charge.

But, it seems, the pineal does rather more than control our circadian rhythms. Drs Pierpaoli and Regelsen, after passionate research, are now sure that it has a very much more important role[17]. No less; it controls our ageing; it is the pineal, they say, which tells our system of endocrine glands to fail, and thus initiate the ageing process. Pierpaoli and Regelsen's work has, we admit, been with populations that are not human; yet mice are very widely used in medical research because they are, in fact, very closely comparable. Their biology is very similar, their body systems and glands work just like ours do, although they may only live for two or three years. By feeding their mice with melatonin, the two doctors showed that the mice lived healthier and longer; not marginally, but very much so.

Not surprisingly, the medical establishment has greeted this work with some scepticism. This is their normal response to anything a bit out of the ordinary in medicine, and probably other scientific disciplines as well. Nevertheless, the work of Pierpoali and Regelsen deserves full attention, and I have found it persuasive and compelling. I think it might be helpful if their findings are summarised.

The relation between melatonin and the immune system is remarkable and decisive. The immune system is our defence against infection, bacteriological, fungal, viral, and against disease in general. As we saw earlier, it consists of T cells and B cells and the macrophages, which consume foreign material. The activity of this defence system is strongly dependent on normal production of melatonin and with ageing, these cells decline in their efficiency. Melatonin seems to prevent this decline; and also to restore and repair the damage done to it by stress. Another interesting thing is that poor sleep reduces the efficiency of the immune system; and the restoration of sleep patterns has a directly useful effect.[18]

The efficient working of the immune system has another vital role to play: it has a seek and destroy facility in the prevention of cancer. This resides especially in the T cells, whose vitality and integrity must be at their very best to detect and destroy the rogue cells, probably always being produced, which, undetected, mean cancer. Work on the hormone-dependent cancers has been especially interesting. We are talking about cancer of the breast, and cancer of the prostate. Melatonin has a regulatory function for our hormone levels, preventing abnormal outputs which affect the risk of cancerous change. Basically, too little, and out of sync, constitutes an increased risk. And the evidence is that melatonin can inhibit the growth of established cancer, by itself, or added to other anti-cancer agents. Worried attention has over the years been directed at the increased vulnerability people have to cancer in high EMF environments (that is, power lines, electric apparatus of all kinds). Melatonin may help to reduce the risk.[19]

The other great scourge of the age is disease of the heart and the arteries: it is an illness more of western high tech civilisation and associated with thoroughly bad eating and smoking more than anything else. The clogging up of our arteries by atheroma is associated with, but not caused by, cholesterol. Arteries already being damaged by free radicals, and by smoking, will clog up quickly when there are high cholesterol levels in the blood. Melatonin has a preventative effect. This is partly perhaps mediated by the thyroid gland, since as I have said, low thyroid output is a major cause of high cholesterol, more than bad eating. With this mechanism, and a second, working through the kidneys, melatonin will reduce blood pressure and lessen the risk of heart attacks and strokes.

There are other aspects of melatonin which may be associated with other beneficial effects, but more study is needed. By enhancing the activity of the immune system, it may help AIDS. It may also help in Alzheimer's disease, especially in association with proper assessment and treatment of low thyroid. Melatonin has been shown to have an effect on the phenomenon of insulin resistance, which is the cause of simpler types of diabetes and obesity. Parkinsonism is another application; many people have responded to melatonin when it has been added to their therapy.[20]

Inevitably, one is asked whether melatonin can improve sexual vigour and interest. Well, it can, but not really directly. The general health and vigour, the maintenance of our glandular system at full operating capacity, the prevention of atherosclerosis, and of course, the anti-ageing effect, all mean improvement in this respect. The enthusiastic activity, reported by the authors, of mice equivalent to a hundred years old, certainly held attention.

We are subjected to, and aged by, endless and unremitting stress. Studies have shown that melatonin will neutralise the harmful effects of stress, directly and by ensuring the glandular system works at its full operating capacity.

We mentioned earlier that melatonin is the hormone of natural sleep. Failing sleep patterns, especially in older people, and those due to stress and anxiety, may be restored by melatonin. All patients have reported improved sleep, using the average dose, 3 mg at night. But it can be used with great effect in the prevention of jet lag, basically speeding up (or slowing down) the body's own adjustments. You take your melatonin before bedtime, at your new destination. If you wake up, repeat the dose.

I believe that, used together with a balanced approach to hormone replacement – male and female HRT, thyroid hormone supplementation, DHEA – melatonin has a decisive role to play in the maintenance of active, vigorous health well beyond our present horizons.

Chapter Eight

The Adrenal Connection

We come now to the second reason for this book. I'm going to tell you about the adrenal glands, what they do, and their connection with thyroid disorders. Some of what I say I will draw from the book, *Safe Uses of Hydrocortisone*, written by William McCormack Jeffries, a gentle, clever and fearless man, who took on the American medical establishment.

The adrenal glands are quite small, about 5 grams each and pyramidal in shape, sitting like little hats on top of each of the kidneys. Small as they are, they have a great deal of work to do, and if for any reason they stopped working, you would be fortunate to survive more than three days. They have an inside, and an outside. The inside is the adrenal medulla, as you can see in the diagram (Figure 12). The adrenal medulla produces adrenaline and noradrenaline. (In the USA, these are called epinephrine and norepinephrine). These are the hormones which allow the body to deal with immediate stress. When you experience a surge of anger, or fear, these hormones are released into the bloodstream, where they mobilise extra blood sugar, increase blood pressure and heart rate. This is the fight or flight reaction.

With this adrenaline surge, you have an immediate increase in energy and muscle strength, your thinking speeds up, and you can cope with huge energy demands to deal with a crisis situation. This capacity is not what concerns us at the moment, however; it is the outside of the adrenal glands, the adrenal cortex, we are most interested in.

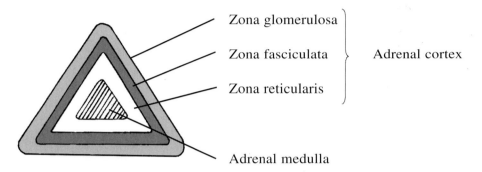

Figure 12. Adrenal cortex and adrenal medulla

The adrenal cortex actually has three layers. The outer layer (zona glomerulosa) produces the mineralocorticoids, represented chiefly by aldosterone. This regulates fluid and electrolyte balance, by promoting the retention of sodium and the loss of potassium in the bloodstream.

The next layer in (zona fasciculata) produces the glucocorticoids, mostly cortisol but also cortisone. The active hormone is cortisol. The glucocorticoids have two main effects: one is the ability to mobilise and form glucose from non sugar sources – fats and proteins – the other is to maintain the muscle tone of the arterial system – vascular tone – which regulates blood pressure. In this way, the glucocorticoids work in the body to protect the body from longer-term, moderate and chronic, stress.

And the last layer (zona reticularis) produces sex hormones and anabolic steroids, that is, androgens and oestrogen. The anabolic steroids are represented by dehydroepiandrosterone (DHEA) and androstendione. The latter can be converted in the fatty tissues of the body to the female sex hormones oestriol, oestrone and oestradiol. Testosterone is also produced. Although it may seem unlikely that both the female and male hormones should be produced together, the interesting thing is that the two hormones, oestradiol and testosterone, are almost identical in structure, differing only in the presence of a hydroxyl (OH) group. Usually these hormones are produced elsewhere, but if normal sources fail, the adrenals can take over. Androgens have the important role of promoting growth and repair of body tissue, especially muscle tissue, as well as their obvious purpose, keeping men male. The zona reticularis layer is weakened by the passage of time and its hormones decline until they are running at a fraction of the output they were in youth.

It is the cortisol production by the adrenals that concerns us in this book. This is the hormone which enables the body to deal with mid- and long-term stress. On our ability to produce this hormone depends our capacity for fighting off the effects of environmental challenges. Injury, illness, deprivation, work or personal stress. Cortisol is the stress buster of the body.

It is produced regularly and constantly, with peaks and troughs. The highest levels are in the morning, declining as the day progresses, and building up again during the small hours. Although the word cortisol may worry you – and we will return to this later – it is a natural substance that we all make and need for our health. In normal health, we make it all our lives, with fairly minimal falling off with age. Problems arise, however, if the adrenal glands go wrong. This may happen in two ways.

The first is overproduction of cortisol. This may occur with overproduction of adrenocorticotrophic hormone (ACTH) by the pituitary. This may be a physiological response to high levels of stress. Stress is used here in its broadest sense; illness, trauma, surgery, or the stress of living in difficult times. This physiological overproduction will not cause a problem generally, since adjustments are automatic; but if there is a hormone producing growth on the pituitary, and it produces too much ACTH all the time, then the overproduction may have damaging effects. A similar hormone-producing tumour (an adenoma) on the adrenal gland itself will cause the same overproduction of cortisol. (This can certainly involve other hormone producing cells of the adrenal, with additional problems.)

The clinical condition so produced is Cushing's disease. Though not especially common, it is seen today more as the result of over-medication with cortisone, which is used in high, therapeutic doses, for a number of conditions including rheumatoid arthritis and related conditions, asthma and chronic allergic disorders. The patient puts on weight, developing a potbelly and rounded moon-face; they develop a thinner, weaker skin, become liable to bruising, and become subject to fluid retention. The treatment is to find the adenoma and surgically remove it, or reduce the amount of cortisone being given.

We are concerned with the opposite end of the scale, which is a great deal more common, but which, in its milder form, may escape detection. In its standard, more severe form, it is called Addison's disease. Thomas Addison described a disease in 1855, where the patient had become chronically ill, with lethargy, loss of appetite, low blood pressure (low enough to cause fainting attacks), hypoglycaemia (extreme sensitivity to lack of carbohydrate and sugars in the diet), a poor response to even mild illness, and a risk of sudden collapse or even death when subject to illness, injury or shock. These unfortunates classically developed a pigmentation or darkening of the skin, especially in skin folds and creases, but also generally. They pursued a steady downhill course, until their death. What struck Addison was that there seemed little to find at post mortem –

except both adrenal glands were taken over by TB bacilli, and consequently not working. Today the adrenals are more likely to be damaged by other processes, most commonly autoimmune diseases; but the principle is the same. There is a steady loss of function, with accumulating symptoms of an illness, which, untreated, will end in death. While gross adrenal failure is not too difficult to diagnose – if it is thought about – it is partial adrenal failure we are concerned about. In the context of this book, I prefer to use the term **low adrenal reserve**.

Signs and Symptoms

Low adrenal reserve is very much more common than fully established Addison's disease, and is affected by the degree of thyroid deficiency also present, and other deficiencies both hormonal and nutritional. Low adrenal reserve is characterised by, firstly, a poor response to stress of any kind. Patients report that they feel ill when stressed, and have to back off at the smallest degree of stress. Illnesses like flu, or a cold, have a devastating effect, lasting longer than they should out of proportion to their severity, and causing much more severe symptoms than would be expected. Patients are chronically hypoglycaemic, and have episodes of faintness and general un-wellness relieved only by sweet tea, or chocolate or a piece of cake. (People often confuse hypoglycaemia, which is episodic low blood sugar, with diabetes. Diabetes is of course quite the reverse; the system loses its ability to control blood sugar, which may rise to abnormally high levels as the result of failure to make enough insulin, or respond to the insulin properly.)

Most patients are both cold and heat sensitive; cold most of the time, they may feel extremely uncomfortable when it's hot and have a cold clammy feel to their skin. There is most commonly present poor absorption of nutrients from food, primarily the result of deficiency of hydrochloric acid in the stomach, and/or a weakness in the production of digestive enzymes, for example the amylases, so the patient may be quite thin. The complexion is pale and almost transparent with a darkness under the eyes most often seen. Pigmentation, especially in skin creases may commonly be noticed. Hair loss will be evident, all over the body, with loss of pubic and underarm hair. Men often lose the hair on their lower legs. Body temperature is low, the skin cold, the Achilles reflexes usually slowed. Patients will often complain of bowel discomfort with wind, diarrhoea and colic; many have been previously diagnosed with the irritable bowel syndrome (IBS). Constant fatigue and exhaustion is always a feature – the batteries running out much too quickly. Fainting and collapse for little cause may also be seen. It will be helpful if you scan the full list of symptoms in Appendix C. It will not escape your attention that many of the symptoms overlap those of hypothyroidism. This should not be surprising, since the thyroid and adrenal glands work together to maintain your metabolism.

You will see from the Appendix that there is a list of signs which the physician will look for if he suspects low adrenal reserve. An especially useful one is Raglan's sign: when the blood pressure is taken, an interesting fact emerges. In normal circumstances when the blood pressure is taken, and the patient is asked to stand up, the systolic (top reading) blood pressure rises 5 or 10 mm of mercury. For example, a sitting blood pressure of say 125/70 will rise to 130/75. But with adrenal weakness the mechanisms for adjusting the blood pressure upward do not work: so that on standing up, the blood pressure may *fall* 5 or 10 mm mercury. This is called **postural hypotension**, and is a cardinal sign of low adrenal reserve. Another useful sign is an unstable pupillary reflex: when a torch is shone into the eye the normal contracting down of the pupil becomes unstable and the pupil opens and closes as if unable to make up its mind.

Diagnostic Tests

It is useful, though not always possible, to confirm the adrenal weakness by blood test. The most obvious test is for the cortisol output from the adrenal glands. Unfortunately, this level is quite extraordinarily variable, depending on the time of day, and the amount of stress present when the test is taken. A white coated physician plunging a needle into an unwilling arm could easily double the serum cortisol within a few moments. A low cortisol level is indeed quite helpful; but a normal level certainly does not rule out low adrenal reserve by any means. One blood test I have found a useful indicator is the serum DHEA sulphate. The adrenals actually produce more DHEA than any other hormone; so a low DHEA level is an indication of weakened adrenal function. However, in patients with low adrenal reserve of long standing there may be an interruption of the biochemical pathway within the adrenal glands where the pro-hormone pregnenolone (see Chapter Seven) is converted to cortisol. When this happens the amount of DHEA may actually build up, with the cortisol showing an abnormal flat response during the day. Extremely valuable is the salivary **adrenal stress index (ASI)**, although, astonishing as it may seem, its worth is often not appreciated by mainstream medicine. Over 24 hours the amount of the two chief adrenal cortex hormones, cortisol and DHEA, is measured. The levels reached, and their relationship to each other, provide valuable information on the amount of stress the adrenals are currently under, and their response to it. A decision can then be made on the adrenal support needed.

A widely used test of adrenal function is the **Synacthen test**. You will remember that ACTH stimulates the adrenals to produce cortisol. Well, if you give ACTH by injection, and then measure in the next 60 minutes the amount of cortisol the adrenals are now making, you have an idea of how responsive and therefore how healthy the adrenals are. Sounds sensible, but the test is greatly troubled by false negatives and will usually only show up adrenals which are really on their last legs. On the whole, as a test it may often not be very helpful.

Another useful investigation is the **24 hour urine test**, which will reveal the breakdown products of cortisol metabolism (the 17 keto-steroids). This can give a valuable 24 hour overview of cortisol production and that of the thyroid also, of course. If the clinical appraisal is not considered sufficient, this urine test may be of great help in convincing your doctor.

Adrenal and Thyroid Connection

We must now consider the adrenal connection to hypothyroidism. The first point to make is a repetition of what I said earlier: if thyroid hormone is not being produced as it should, *nothing* works properly – including of course the adrenal glands. And this situation is compounded by the fact that low thyroid output is a stress inducing situation. To enable the system to cope with low thyroid output, the adrenals are obliged to produce an increased level of cortisol. This may work well, for a considerable period of time, if the thyroid deficiency isn't too bad. But it slowly worsens and the adrenals are called upon to further compensate for the stress this produces. Eventually, of course, the adrenals begin to cope less well; and the continued strain causes adrenal exhaustion. The syndrome of low adrenal reserve is now present.

Clearly the drift into this situation is dependent on a number of factors. Your general health, nutrition, lifestyle and other stresses all play a part. The length of time the thyroid problem has gone on for – and how badly. The cause of the deficiency: I have found radioactive iodine or surgery to the thyroid a particular problem for the adrenal glands. Another very real problem, of course, is incorrect treatment. Supplementary thyroid hormone may of itself cause stress if the system cannot cope with it; it is possible to trigger a thyroid/adrenal crisis and collapse using the wrong sort of dose, and ignoring the necessity of providing adrenal support – that is, ensuring the adrenal glands *can* cope with the strain. Indeed, it is possible by using thyroxine, when the patient cannot convert it properly, to cause a full Addisonian crisis, which may be fatal.

We saw earlier that the thyroid hormones have to be processed in the body to work; the chief one, thyroxine (T4) has to be converted into the active thyroid hormone tri-iodothyronine (T3), under the action of the 5'-deiodinase enzymes. With a low adrenal reserve this reaction doesn't proceed as it should, and the body may become toxic with unused and unusable T4. The problem doesn't end there; the T3 has to be taken up by the receptors within the cell wall, to be passed into the cell. This uptake is degraded in adrenal insufficiency; the receptors become dormant or may disappear or may become resistant. In this situation, even if T3 is available, the system can become toxic if it cannot be used properly. You can see how desperately important the adrenal glands are, and equally how important it is to provide adrenal support when low adrenal reserve is present. I must tell you now that the failure of thyroid supplementation to restore normal health may well be largely down to the adrenal problem. This is scarcely ever considered by physicians since they do not recognise low adrenal reserve, and may even miss the diagnosis of established Addison's disease.

Thousands of people suffering from hypothyroidism are never quite well since, using the blood tests as a guide only, the endocrinologists with few exceptions oblige their patients to lurch from one dose to another. The patients may have windows of feeling better, but may feel either under-active, or toxic for much of the time. The great sadness is that when they say to their doctor, 'Look, I really don't feel right,', they will be told, since the blood tests show that they are at the correct levels, they *must* therefore be right and perfectly well – whatever they may say. The patient is then probably offered Prozac (or other antidepressant), or counselling, or becomes labelled a 'heart-sink' patient, and you can see now why the blood tests may be completely misleading. If the thyroid supplementation *isn't being used properly* and is not being processed into the tissues, it will cause the blood levels to be normal, or even raised. In this situation, which is likely to affect all hypothyroid sufferers sooner or later, if this is not taken account of the patient will *never* be well. Along with a number of other workers in this field, I have pointed this out many times to the deaf ears of the establishment. Whatever you may be told, adrenal insufficiency in thyroid disorders is very common indeed and should always be considered at the onset of treatment. Failure to respond to thyroid supplementation, or actually feeling less well, is likely more often than not to involve the low adrenal reserve syndrome. So let us now look at how we can keep our adrenals in optimum health and how to provide support when there is damage.

Adrenal Stress Management

Adrenal stress management requires that everything possible is done to reduce the cause of adrenal stress. Firstly, we must reduce external stress. This implies **lifestyle changes**, which may be practical only to a limited degree. Avoidance of emotional, work, or financial stress is obvious, but may be a counsel of perfection. Cutting down our exposure to television and computer screens is also helpful.

It means going to bed early, by 10 pm (dammit), to follow our natural biorhythms (when melatonin switches our system off). Night time, especially just before waking, is when most cortisol production happens, so when we wake in the morning we have the cortisol required for the day, which will slowly tail off and then be replenished when we go to sleep again. It is essential that help is given if there is a real problem with sleeping, and melatonin and valerian can be of use here.

Then there are mental ways of reducing stress. Yoga, or meditation, bio-feedback comes into this; listening to music, laughter, are to be considered also – watch your favourite comedy programme. *Dad's Army* does wonders for me...

Exercise is another important factor – walking especially. Even half an hour a day, perhaps broken into 10 minute slots, will help. And it quietens the mind.

We now have to consider three treatment options. The first is to provide all the nutrients the adrenal glands need to work properly.

Diet

You should eat a proper, healthful, organic diet, without the stress of chemical or toxic exposure and without food intolerances or allergies. The avoidance of long periods of fasting is desirable – one should eat perhaps four times a day. There are certain foodstuffs which can help the adrenal glands and these are: watercress, parsley, slippery elm, yucca, coconut oil/milk, and royal jelly. Sufficient **potassium** is quite necessary, and a correct ratio with **salt** (sodium) is important; ideally, the ratio should be 5 of potassium to 1 of salt. Potassium is found, as we know, in bananas; but also in fresh vegetables and fruit. Avocados are another good source, and so are potatoes. Coffee, smoking and other stimulants are to be avoided; people with adrenal insufficiency can be strikingly intolerant of even small amounts of alcohol. Refined carbohydrates, especially processed, such as bread, cakes and sugar, should be sharply reduced.

Most important is **vitamin C**, required for the enzyme processes throughout the complex adrenal cascade. The turnover of vitamin C is always increased in times of stress. It is required in substantial doses, divided over the day: no less than 2 grams per day, and may be up to 10 grams. Should it cause indigestion or looseness of the bowel, you should modify the intake accordingly. Some people have delicate stomachs and will benefit from buffered vitamin C.

Equally important is **vitamin B$_5$** (pantothenic acid); a deficiency is linked with loss of adrenal function and atrophy. The many conversions in the adrenal cascade require the vitamin as a cofactor in these reactions. A diet of whole grains, legumes, cauliflower, broccoli, salmon, liver, sweet potatoes and tomatoes will provide B$_5$. Otherwise 100-500 micrograms (mcg) daily may be given. Other essential nutrients are **liquorice**, which in the form of the root, tablets (2 or 3 a day, 5-15 milligrams or mg), or tincture, prolongs the effectiveness of cortisone by inhibiting the enzymes that break it down. Chinese and Siberian **ginseng** (these belong to a group of nutritional supplements called adaptogens) have a supportive role in biological processes. **Essential fatty acids** are also required, most especially the omega-3 group, (since we tend to have too much of omega-6 and omega-9). These come from fish oils, flax and hemp seed oils. Other nutrients include **vitamin B$_6$** (50-100 mcg), **coenzyme Q10**, and the elemental minerals **manganese** (4 mg), **magnesium** (250-500 mg), **zinc** (20-30 mg) or elemental zinc (10 mg) and **chromium** (120 mcg), **copper** (1 mg), and **freeform flavonoids** (500 mg) should also be part of the supplement regime. All these supplements can be added to your daily diet.

Adrenal Support

The second option is the provision of **glandular concentrate** supplementation. This is normally prepared from specially processed bovine adrenal concentrates.

One example is from Nutri Ltd who produce a standard preparation of 80 mg of concentrate, another of 221 mg concentrate together with vitamins and minerals. Nutri-Meds is another supplier, and like Nutri Ltd, may be accessed by phone or online (contact details are at the back of the book). The important fact about these preparations is that they contain all the adrenal hormones, and the enzymes to make them, so that they act synergistically with your own adrenals, and so help in the recovery of adrenal function. Once the adrenals are coming on line in this way, it becomes possible to introduce the thyroid supplementation, usually within two or three weeks, in the way I describe shortly. It is usually necessary to keep the adrenal support going for several months, after which it can be tailed off. Commonly, somewhere between two and four tablets are needed, building up from one before food in the morning, and the remainder before 1 pm, the final dose depending on how exhausted the adrenal glands are.

Another approach is to support the adrenal cascade directly. This will require: **pregnenolone** (30 mg), or **DHEA** (25 mg), or **7-keto DHEA** (25 mg); all taken first thing in the morning. (If there is a blockage to cortisol manufacture at the 17-OH pregnenolone level, then biotin should be taken to maintain enzymatic production such as the 21-hydroxylase enzyme.) These supplements are considered nutrients in the USA and may be obtained as such, but require a prescription in the UK.

Where adrenal function is very badly compromised, and the natural glandular concentrate is not going to be enough, there are further options, which I shall explain in a moment. But first, I want to explain a little more about the thyroid and adrenal relationship.

Bringing the metabolism back in line with thyroid hormone may actually cause adrenal stress, and there may be a further, if temporary, loss of adrenal function.

This will interfere with processing and uptake of the thyroid hormone, which may then build up, unused, and create a toxic effect. This has been called T4 toxicosis, and symptoms include feeling generally unwell, perhaps as if hyped, with a rapid heart rate and even chest pain similar to angina. The thyroid supplementation should be stopped, adrenal support put in place, and then after an interval the thyroid support can be started again. (This is described in detail below.)

A problem often arises when those of us with low thyroid seek advice, and it becomes clear that low adrenal reserve is at least half the problem. The amount of thyroid hormone replacement, usually thyroxine, has been increased, either with very little benefit, or actually worsening the situation. If the adrenal support is then given, it has the effect of so much improving thyroid uptake and processing, that in a day or so, you actually become truly thyrotoxic, with palpitations, tremor, even a temperature. To deal with this situation low cunning is needed. The thyroxine must be stopped for 5-10 days to allow it to run down somewhat. (Remember that it has an eight day half life in the system, so this can be quite a slow process.) After these few days, natural adrenal glandular support is introduced, at low dose – even half a tablet – and after a few days without any problems of apparent overdose, the adrenal support can then be increased to one, and later more if required. At some point, usually within a week, the thyroid hormone can be restarted at half the original dose. All the time you have to monitor pulse and temperature, on a daily basis, morning and evening, and then be prepared to adjust the thyroid hormone dose up or down as seems necessary. A rapid rise of pulse, perhaps into the 90s per minute or a *sudden* rise of temperature to apparently normal levels, is likely to mean that the thyroid supplementation is too much and should be reduced or stopped for a day or so. Low adrenal reserve commonly means that as the day progresses, cortisol particularly becomes exhausted, and with it thyroid uptake and processing. Hence as the day goes on, one can feel more tired (more so than one should) than in the morning, and the pulse and temperature will show this by dropping. It is helpful to take the temperature and pulse in the evening (say 9 or 10 o'clock), to monitor the adrenal status. If the adrenal glands are becoming exhausted the temperature will drop and the pulse rate may do so as well. This regime is effective for the majority of people with adrenal and thyroid dysfunction. Moreover, it can be used safely with the minimum of medical supervision, since we are using food supplements rather than synthetic preparations.

Where the adrenal support needs to be at a higher level, manufactured prescription hydrocortisone has to be used. It is provided as tablets of hydrocortisone B.P. (British Pharmacopia) 10 mg.

The guiding principle is to provide adrenal support *physiologically*. This means that the amount of supplementation is comparable to the amount actually produced by the body itself in the normal healthy state. The distinction between physiological dosage and therapeutic dosage is crucial to understand. A therapeutic dose is in excess of the natural production (or physiological) dose, and will inevitably suppress the natural production.

The natural output of hydrocortisone is actually variable and may be as much as 200 mg daily under stress and 40-60 mg in a normal resting state. Obviously then, a dose significantly greater than 40 mg daily will tend to take over the adrenal production of cortisone, and the adrenal glands could shut down completely. But it must be said at once, so long as this suppression doesn't last too long, the adrenals will pick themselves up again, and restart producing the necessary cortisol for themselves as before. One spectre that gibbers in the sight of many physicians is this adrenal suppression. It is only temporary unless very prolonged; and the adrenals will resume normal function *as far as they are able* when supplementation is discontinued. The problem is of course they may not come back to normal until the thyroid/adrenal deficiency has been adequately treated for long enough. A physiological replacement level would therefore be 15 or 20 mg daily, required until the patient is making a satisfactory response to the treatment as a whole.

I want to hammer home the distinction between *physiological* cortisone replacement, which may be quite essential to the overall management of thyroid/adrenal insufficiency, and *therapeutic* cortisone dosage. It was found as far back as 1948, that supra-normal dosage of cortisone had remarkable benefits on people crippled with rheumatoid arthritis and related collagen disorders – systemic sclerosis, systemic lupus erythematosus – and people invalided with intractable asthma, together with other, up to then, untreatable conditions. The downside to the miraculous recoveries cortisone brought to people's lives, were side effects. They were the same as I mentioned in relation to Cushing's syndrome; but in addition there was a risk of sudden death after operations or major trauma, with a generally reduced ability to deal with infection. This turned out to be due to adrenal suppression by the high doses of cortisone; when called to respond in a high-challenge situation the adrenal glands were unable to do so, and the patient slipped into irreversible surgical shock and died.

When this became widely known cortisone was used with a great deal more care; doses were reduced and given over a limited time interval, and when the cortisone was stopped, it was done gradually so that the adrenals could pick up and revert to normal activity. As it does, the pendulum has now swung very far the other way, and in the minds of patients and doctors alike, there is a deep horror and aversion to the use of cortisone in any context whatsoever. This extreme hostility to the use of cortisone, even its very mention, by physicians and their patients is greatly to be deplored and is one important reason why the management of thyroid insufficiency is in such a parlous state and so misunderstood and misused. I must emphasise again, that the use of low dosage, that is *physiological* dosage, of cortisone, is not only perfectly safe in restoring proper adrenal response, but is often absolutely essential. Along with many of my American colleagues, I have been the subject of much ill-informed criticism of this view, based on a prejudice arising from its previous history of improper use. But facts are facts and it is essential that physicians and patients alike rethink the whole problem. Two quotations from the great physician McCormack Jeffries are really quite relevant.

'Cortisol is a normal hormone, essential for life.'

'Most physicians today are under the impression that *any* dosage of cortisol can produce side effects that occur with any excessive doses.'

Undoubtedly for the clinician, the replacement of choice is hydrocortisone, since this, though synthetically produced, is identical to naturally produced cortisone. But, the initial approach has to be restrained and cautious, and the lowest possible dose given at the start. I found that one quarter of a 10 mg tablet of hydrocortisone (that is, 2.5 mg) is an excellent starting point.

Once the hydrocortisone is started the full support dose is now built up to effective levels over two or three weeks. The quarter tablet a day is increased to a quarter tablet twice a day; then after a few days, 3 times a day and up to a quarter four times a day, spread out throughout the waking day. The reason for this is that it is not stored by the body and gets rapidly used; two or three hours will see it pretty well used up completely. Since a smooth level of support is desirable, the dose does need to be spread out. The final dose is usually 20 mg daily, that is half a tablet four times a day; but careful adjustment relating to the response may take the dose to 25 mg or 30 mg daily, exceptionally even 40 mg. These higher doses are related more to absorption in the stomach than to deficiency, but low adrenal reserve reaching Addisonian levels may make such doses necessary.

If hydrocortisone has a disadvantage, it is the fact that it needs to be given four times a day to be fully effective. Some patients do as well, or better, on the widely used synthetic derivative, prednisolone. The equivalent dose of 20 mg of hydrocortisone is 5 mg of prednisolone, which may be increased up to 7.5 mg. This needs to be given only once a day, most commonly in the morning, since it remains active in the system for about 24 hours. Because prednisolone can irritate the stomach on occasion, it is usually given in an enteric coated version called Deltacortril; and if given with food the risk of gastric irritation is further minimised.

Where there is considerable electrolyte imbalance, it is sometimes useful also to prescribe a mineralocorticoid, and the most widely used is fludrocortisone or Florinef, in doses of 0.1 mg once or twice a day. This may further improve the adrenal response when given together with the glucocorticoids, hydrocortisone or prednisolone. There are other synthetic cortisones available, but in general they shouldn't prove necessary.

The length of time necessary to provide adrenal support is really very variable. My normal practice has usually been to obtain the best result with thyroid and adrenal support, and after six or eight weeks, start to tail off the cortisone supplement. If there is no adverse result it may then be stopped – taking, say, four weeks in the process. Sometimes the patient starts to lose ground; and you then have the choice of replacing it with a glandular concentrate for a longer period or restarting the cortisone, and in another eight weeks or so another attempt to tail it off is made. Sometimes, the adrenals have been so badly hit that the adrenal support may be required for months, and if the adrenal glands never fully recover, for a more indefinite time. Again, I emphasise that if adrenal support *is* required, it must be given for as long as it takes; there is no risk to this since one is simply restoring the situation to normal, in the same way, and for the same reason, that thyroid support may have to be given indefinitely.

To summarise the indications where adrenal support may be needed, we may say:

1. Where an abnormally low DHEA and an abnormally high cortisol show adrenal stress, or abnormally low cortisol and DHEA blood test shows weak adrenal function.

2. Many symptoms, and clinical signs, notably postural hypotension, suggest weak adrenal response.

3. The thyroid deficiency state has been present some considerable time and is getting worse.

4. Previous treatment with thyroxine has been unsuccessful or even worsened the situation.

5. There has been thyroid surgery or radioactive iodine ablation.

6. Thyroid blood tests are normal but the patient is clinically hypothyroid.

7. Previous major surgery or trauma/shock from an accident or life event.

Chapter Nine

Hypothyroidism – The Treatment

As I said at the start of the book, the first recorded successful treatment of thyroid deficiency was that due to the physician Murray in 1898. The two ladies with advanced hypothyroidism I mentioned in the Introduction, were given thyroid extract. This was crushed animal thyroid and fairly unpleasant. But both ladies were cured. Soon, the unpalatable extract was dehydrated and compressed into tablet form and is still very successfully in use today. I personally can testify to its extraordinary efficacy. From the time of Murray, although understanding of the mechanisms of thyroid failure is now more complete, for which Broda Barnes and John Lowe in the USA must be especially thanked, the treatment has not progressed very much. Indeed, most of the evidence suggests that patients are not doing as well as they used to.

The first problem lies in diagnosis. Although hypothyroidism is more common than it used to be, it is less often diagnosed. A leading expert has it that 1 in 20 people may develop hypothyroidism. I think he is terribly wrong; it seems to me that the figure is much more like 1 in 3 or 4.[1,2,3] Hypothyroidism is just a bit too obvious, too common; it is more fashionable to find a more complex diagnosis, or to fall back on stress or depression. Before 1960, the diagnosis was made on clinical grounds: you looked and listened. The advent of blood tests has made cowards of us all. I have been told so many times that the GP, suspecting hypothyroidism, has done the standard blood test; it comes back 'in the normal range', and the doctor then dismisses the diagnosis, in spite of glaring physical evidence to the contrary. The patient may then demand referral to the local consultant endocrinologist. There are some wonderful exceptions, but for the most part having done some more tests, he will come to the same conclusion. Many are actually unpleasant and unkind, and I have been told too often that the luckless patient has been reduced to tears for wasting their time. Patients will be told they are suffering from stress, not getting enough sleep, not dressing warmly enough, or are simply depressed – anything that will explain the contradiction between the symptoms & signs, and the blood test result.

One such consultant, typical of many, was actually brave enough to put his thoughts into print. He wrote a press release in the British Thyroid Foundation Newsletter. Quote. 'The stresses and strains of modern life, however, commonly cause similar symptoms and when the effect of our miserable weather is added, it is not surprising that many people are convinced that their thyroid gland is abnormal, even when it is not.' He continued, 'Pity the poor endocrinologist'. I have paraphrased the rest.

> 'You're tired? So are we all. Get to bed early.'
> 'You're overweight? Eat better and more carefully.'
> 'You're cold? Wear a thicker pullover.'
> 'You're depressed? Empty nest syndrome, my dear.'
> 'Periods heavy? Often are at your age.'

And so on and so on… Thanks to this kind of uncaring approach, hundreds and hundreds of patients are condemned to endless worsening ill-health, with a good chance of a premature death. So that is why so many patients with hypothyroidism remain ill – they don't get diagnosed in the first place.

If they *are* diagnosed, the simplistic approach may well mean that fewer than half ever enjoy a return to good health. What we must now do is to consider the treatment options that *are* available, if you are lucky enough to be diagnosed and treated by an informed and sympathetic doctor.

Treatment has to be considered at various levels and the keynote is for a holistic approach. Holistic means considering the patient as a whole, not just separate aspects of a patient's illness. So we will make a list.

Environmental hazards. Take out of your environment all the toxins and poisons that may have damaged your thyroid in the first place. Okay, I am not going to ask you to stop your morning coffee or your glass of wine with dinner; but too much of anything is a *bad thing*. I need to be more severe about smoking. So keep it all within bounds. Check what medicines you are already having to see what can be done to reduce or stop them where practical. For example, medicines like barbiturates, lithium and amiodarone are known to affect thyroid function. (Lithium must be stopped under medical supervision.) Remember what we said about fluoride. Find out if your water is fluoridated; if it is, filter it or drink bottled water (preferably from glass bottles). Those of vegetarian persuasion should be reminded that cabbages and cauliflowers and sprouts (the brassicas) contain thiouracil, which slows down thyroid hormone production. The damaging effect of chemicals in our foodstuffs, the preservatives, the E numbers, the packaging, is something we may not always wish to think about. Phthalate esters, which comprise most plastic wrappings, are poisonous in several respects, not least to our thyroids. The bottom line is, wherever you can, try and eat as organically as possible. We are surrounded by noxious chemicals in the very air we breathe – every source must be reduced as far as possible.

Adequate nutritional supplementation. While eating well and sensibly, and avoiding junk food are obvious precautions, hypothyroidism may have been partly the result of poor absorption of vital minerals and vitamins, compounding the problem. Almost certainly, there should be supplementation of all of these. Iodine, if deficient, should be added, but remember, although iodine makes the thyroid hormone actually do the work, too much will cause thyroid suppression. Minerals are very important and a multi-mineral preparation is clearly desirable. Vitamins are equally important, especially B_{12} if pernicious anaemia is present. Vitamin C has a number of benefits in the system.[4, 5] In particular, as we know, it is an antioxidant and is essential in the prevention of scurvy. But it also acts as an adrenal support (which is why common cold remedies contain vitamin C), so that a gram or two a day can only be beneficial. Other vitamins may be close to their minimum required levels and supplementation of them is a must. In passing, there has been pressure from doctors who should know better, that vitamin C isn't as good for you as was previously thought and sadly there seems to be a trend against natural medicines, vitamins and minerals in current medical thinking. Sometimes, simply providing the right nutrients makes a decisive difference.

Provision of adrenal support. In Chapter Eight I pointed out that anyone with thyroid deficiency over a period of time, especially if it is more than mild, is likely to have their deficiency accompanied and complicated by the low adrenal reserve syndrome. If this is not dealt with *before* providing thyroid supplementation, response may be disappointing, and there is a risk of a thyroid crisis. This occurs when the system becomes overwhelmed with thyroid replacement from the medication, which it is unable to deal with, and the patient may have violent palpitations, headaches or collapse. The obvious difficulty lies in knowing whether adrenal support is required. Well, the difficulty is more imaginary than real. First, the history of the symptoms, the postural hypotension, the fainting attacks, the digestive upsets and the other problems I mentioned in the last chapter, along with possible pointers from a blood test, are likely to make low adrenal reserve a strong possibility. Secondly, if there *is* any doubt, initial support *must* be given since there are real problems if it *is* needed and *not* given. Thirdly, prescribed in the way I discussed earlier, there is no risk, since the amount of adrenal support is physiological. This means, even if it isn't necessary, no damage is done, no risks are taken and it can be withdrawn whenever thought appropriate.

Exercise. Thyroid health, much like our health generally, of course, requires proper exercise. The importance of daily exercise cannot be overstated; start with gentle stretching first thing in the morning to get the blood flowing through the endocrine glands. You need to walk perhaps more often than you do now, take the stairs, do aerobic exercise when you can. People with weak thyroids are often found in the gym because the exercise stimulates their thyroid function and metabolism.

Now, there is one thing I would like to say before going deeper into the treatment, and it may sound slightly negative, although that is not the intention. Because most of you will in actual fact have been ill for some time before seeking help or being treated, there will have been certain changes in the body, which may never be quite reversed. Two reasons: one, the ageing process will have been in action over this time; and two, as you are replacing missing hormones and nutrients, it can never be just how the body would do it, and so there will be off days – but not many. That said, we now need to look first at the raw materials the thyroid needs in our diet.

We need protein for the amino acid **phenylalanine** – wheat, oats, meat, poultry, fish, eggs, cheese, pulses and nuts. Some 2 ounces a day is an average requirement. **Tyrosine** supplements may be added if the diet is short of sufficient protein, 500 milligrams (mg) to 2 grams (g) daily.

Iodine foodstuffs are required in moderation: fish and seafood contain the most and then fruit and vegetables. Where required it can be taken daily in the form of kelp tablets – 100 mg of kelp provides 150 micrograms (mcg) of iodine.

Selenium is found in offal, meats, fish, shellfish, dairy products, citrus fruit, avocado pears and whole grains. A very good source is brazil nuts. If supplementation is required you will need 200 mcg daily but since synthetic forms of selenium are not very well absorbed, it is preferable to ensure a good supply in your diet.

Other trace substances are required in the manufacture and processing of thyroid hormones and I have listed the daily amounts below.

Vitamins

A – 800 iu

B Complex: high strength

(B_1, B_2, B_3, B_6, B_{12}, Folate)

C – 1 to 2 g

E – 400 to 800 iu

D – 15 mcg

Minerals

Manganese – 4 mg

Calcium – 1000 to 1500 mg

Magnesium – 300 mg

Zinc – 15 to 20 mg

Chromium – 120 mcg

Iron – 15 mg

Copper – 2 mg

Flavonoids, Carotenoids & CoEnzyme Q10 are also required.

All these essential nutrients can be provided in thyroid support supplements (for example Nutri's Thyro Complex) or taken separately.

Claims have been made that coconut oil is supportive of a weakened metabolism and it may well be helpful.

As I have said, some things shouldn't be eaten or should be avoided in large quantities and these are called **goitrogenic** foods. The brassicas – cabbage, brussel sprouts – contain thiouracil which inhibits the actual manufacture of thyroid hormone; others are turnips, cassava, pine nuts, mustard, peanuts and millet. Soya, due to the high levels of phyto-oestrogens. Our *British cuppa* contains **fluoride** (the tea plant likes fluoride rich soils) and perhaps some of us should remember this when calling for our tenth cup.

We must now turn our attention to the treatment of the thyroid deficiency state. Having put in place the adrenal support if needed, it is now safe to provide the thyroid support, and we can be sure that it is actually going to work. Although there are several options available, you are most likely to be offered only one – if you can convince the doctor in charge of your need. If you can't, all is not lost; you can take control of your own health.

The use of thyroxine for hypothyroidism is considered by most physicians to be the only treatment on the table. But this is very far from the case. When Murray first treated his patients, he used raw sheep thyroid sandwiches. The patients got better, it's true, and a new and wonderful chapter opened in the annals of medicine, but for some reason there was a distinct lack of patient compliance. At length, the thyroid was dried and processed into tablets, which everybody preferred. And they all got better just the same. We still use the principle today in thyroid glandular concentrate, and desiccated thyroid.

Where the thyroid has been damaged in some way, and cannot be expected to recover full function, we can turn to the earliest days of thyroid treatment, and the use of processed **glandular concentrates**. Extremely useful is whole glandular bovine or porcine thyroid concentrate, which contains 130 mg of raw thyroid concentrate. Nutri-Meds in the USA, and Nutri Ltd in the UK prepare these products, which are designated as dietary supplements and so do not require a prescription, although they do have to be recommended by a healthcare practitioner. The dosage levels may be largely set by the patient: monitoring symptoms, temperature and pulse should enable the correct dose to be arrived at. The dose is normally 1 or 2 tablets daily with food, usually in the morning; this may be increased after a few months to 3 or 4. All the time you must monitor your waking and evening temperature and pulse to assess your physical response, making a note of how you feel.

The next treatment option is the use of **natural desiccated thyroid**. Many of you reading this are aware that I have been a keen protagonist of natural thyroid for some 25 years, along with a number of other workers in the field, taking my lead from Broda Barnes, Jacques Hertoghe and more recently John Lowe. We prefer it because it works better than synthetic thyroid, which after all is the most important thing. Patients almost always prefer it, because they actually feel better on the natural rather than the synthetic; and it should go without saying that the body responds better to natural molecules than synthetic ones. (It *should* go without saying, but it doesn't among establishment endocrinologists, who sadly do not always actually listen to what the patient is telling them.) In fact, natural thyroid has been used since the inception of thyroid treatment, and so has a 100 year history of safe use in clinical practice. It is widely used in the USA and increasingly in the UK.

It is objected to on several specious grounds. Some doctors, who really should know better, point to the risk of BSE. Firstly, natural thyroid is made in the USA, where the strictest controls are undertaken to ensure there is no BSE; and secondly, most comes from pigs, who don't get it anyway. And pig thyroid is very close to our own thyroid, with all the hormones in the right balance, which has to be better than one or two artificial hormones. Additionally, there is likelihood of improved absorption of the natural product, and improved biochemical processing. Widely available in the USA, in England it is obtained by special order – where a prescription and a letter are required – from certain chemists. Most doctors are amazed that in England it was widely used until 1985, when it became no longer economical to manufacture. The medical establishment widely put it about that the synthetic preparation (which was very much cheaper) was far better since the amount of thyroid hormone was more precise. This quite ignores the fact that since thyroid production in the body is variable anyway, it doesn't matter if the dose is not quite precise. Actually the amount of thyroid hormone in the natural preparations *is* precisely controlled, and by contrast the American synthetic thyroxine preparation Synthroid has been under a dark cloud over recent years.[6]

The fact remains that natural desiccated thyroid USP (Armour is the most popular) is preferred by patients and works better than synthetic thyroxine and is therefore the treatment of choice. Forest Pharmaceuticals in the USA, who manufacture Armour, have a website which updates patients and doctors alike of all the most recent research, answering many thousands of queries. The sympathetic and very well informed Dr Joseph Mercola plays a major role in this and further information is freely available from Mary Shomon's and Thyroid UK's sites (see Appendix D).

The use of natural thyroid follows the same general lines of treatment as with the synthetic. Adrenal support is put in place first if required, and then the natural thyroid should be started. The tablets are in ½, 1 or 2 grains, which are older measures, sadly driven out of this country's chemists by decimalisation. (A rough equivalent is that 1 grain, which is a 60 mg tablet = 39 mcg of T4 and 9 mcg of T3.) It makes sense to start with ½ grain but usually this can be increased to 1 grain within a week or so. After 10 to 14 days, the dose may be reviewed and increased in increments of ½ grain up to probably no more than 2 grains, when a period of several weeks may elapse for the response to stabilise, still, of course, under careful self-monitoring. At this time the dose can be reviewed and changed up or down according to need.

The use of **thyroxine** (called Eltroxin in UK, and Synthroid in USA) is considered by most physicians to be the only treatment on the table. A number of generic brands are now available, but some patients and doctors have found they lack consistent efficacy. It comes as tiny white tablets of 25, 50 and 100 micrograms (mcg). It is always sensible to start with the lowest dose, especially in the elderly; so common practice is to start with 25 mcg. This may be increased in increments, up to a dose regarded as standard of 100 mcg. At this point most physicians stay their hand, and the patient may have to remain on this dose until kingdom come, with any changes of dose decided by blood test exclusively, little regard often being paid to how the patient actually feels. The problem with this is that it takes no account of low adrenal reserve or conversion blocks, or receptor uptake insufficiency. Also, this is not the way nature does it. As we saw earlier, thyroid hormone is 80% thyroxine, 17% tri-iodothyronine, and the remainder T2 and T1. The fact that patients with non-severe thyroid sufficiency manage on T4 alone is no credit to the physicians. If the condition is not too far advanced or of too long standing, all the thyroxine (T4) will be converted to tertroxin (T3) and used with consequent patient benefit. Sadly, many endocrinologists refuse to accept that supplementing thyroid hormone *the way nature does it* is necessary or desirable, mostly on the grounds that they know best. I must tell you now that, except for mild early cases, this is not the best way to provide thyroid supplementation.

The more serious thyroid deficiency will respond only poorly to this regime, since it takes no account of the adrenal connection, conversion block, or receptor uptake resistance. The patient may feel an initial benefit, but within days or weeks this may wear off; or the patient may soon start to become aware of tremors and palpitations. The blood test may well show the presence of too much thyroid in the blood – since it is not being used – and the dose will be reduced. This makes the side effects better but the exhaustion and fluid retention and all the other symptoms will still be there, poorly relieved, if at all. It is this situation that I found in about 70% of the patients (already on treatment) I saw for the first time. The conclusion is obvious: for the very large number of patients, thyroxine may only work very poorly or not at all for the reasons we discussed. But even if these problems are dealt with the response may still be disappointing. So we need to consider other options.

The first is to understand that the 5'-deiodinase enzymes carrying out the T4 $\rightarrow$ T3 conversion may be quite deficient or not even work at all. The build up of unused T4 is then inevitable, and within a relatively short time there may be toxic levels present with palpitations, a general lack of well-being, stomach upsets and so on. It may well be quite impossible to predict that this is going to happen, which is why it is necessary to start the treatment in a standard way, the patient doing the monitoring on a daily basis: pulse and temperature, am and pm, and perhaps something like a 1 to 10 feel good factor, all written down daily. If symptoms occur and things are not right, the thyroxine is discontinued, but everything else remains in place, including the adrenal support. When the coast is clear, say in 7 to 10 days, one or two alternatives may now be used. Using the thyroid supplementation obtainable from your doctor on prescription, we may now use the already converted thyroid hormone, the **liothyronine (T3)**. This is marketed in the UK as Tertroxin, 20 mcg tablets and in the USA as Cytomel, 25 mcg tablets.

The T3 is the active thyroid hormone that actually does the work of controlling metabolism. It has two important differences from thyroxine. First, it is rapidly metabolised, having a half-life of about 8 hours, unlike thyroxine, which is more like 8 days. So the blood levels decline rapidly at first and then more slowly, but *some* remains for some time. In practical terms though, there is pretty well no T3 left worth talking about after 24 hours or so. This is unlike T4, which takes time to build up its levels in the bloodstream and 3 or 4 weeks at least for the amount in the blood to drop below a therapeutically effective level. This means that T3 works a good deal quicker than T4.

The second difference is that microgram for microgram T3 is a good deal more powerful than thyroxine; something like five times stronger. So the amount given is proportionately less; and in general 20 mcg of T3 is considered the equivalent to 100 mcg of T4.

Start the dose of T3 at ½ x 20 mcg tablet daily, certainly before midday. After five days or so, the dose may be increased subject to your careful monitoring. Authorities are undecided as to whether the dose is better split into two, or given all at once in the morning; best, probably to decide yourself – but evening is not a good time since then it is likely to interfere with sleep.

As time goes on the overall dose may be increased, allowing plenty of time to decide how it is all going, by small increments: say, ½ a tablet at a time. After decided improvement and probably not sooner than eight weeks, it may be possible to substitute T4 for at least one dose of T3, because the conversion problem may be easing. It is perfectly possible to stay on T3 alone, permanently, and many patients have to. The important thing is to keep a flexible approach and not be afraid to experiment; so long as it is all monitored, then you can be sure of what is doing what. The ultimate dose should be whatever suits you best; it may be, for example, ½ T3 and ½T4, or ¾ of one and ¼ of the other, or any variation that works.

Doctor Blanchard in the USA recommends that the proportion of T3 to T4 is at its most satisfactory if the patient is provided with 98% of T4 to 2% of T3. As far as I know, however, this regime has not gained general acceptance.

There are a number of factors which can affect the overall need for thyroid supplementation. One, of course, is the change in status of your own thyroid. With the whole system reverting to normal on treatment, it happens that pituitary control and thyroid response may improve, making thyroid supplementation less necessary or sometimes even unnecessary altogether. The second, is the reverse: whatever process is damaging the thyroid, for example autoimmune disease, it continues and the natural output continues to fall away making an increase of thyroid supplementation necessary.

There is the season factor. Basically, the colder the external temperature is, the more heat the body needs to compensate, and therefore metabolism has to be increased – so more thyroid hormone has to be made. And if it cannot be increased internally, then extra has to be provided. The reverse obviously applies in hot weather and in hot climates. I have taught all my patients to be prepared to increase their thyroid supplementation in the winter and reduce it in the summer. In any event you must keep an open and flexible approach to your dosage, since your needs may vary from day to day or week to week for no apparent reason. If you listen to what your body is telling you and make adjustments accordingly, you will derive the fullest benefit from your supplementation.

There may also be changes in natural output as a result of illness, or major life events. While, once the dose is settled on, the self-monitoring is not so much required, nevertheless a change in well-being should encourage you to pick up your thermometer again.

I want to introduce a note of comfort here. The dose can go wrong in either of two ways:

1. You can have too little. Then symptoms start to creep back, temperature and pulse fall, and the penny should drop.

2. You can also have too much. Let me say at once, that an overdose will occur quite slowly but should be obvious from symptoms and pulse and temperature changes quite soon. The establishment medical approach is to make a great deal of noise about the dangers of overdose. There are indeed dangers of overdose, but it has to be quite substantial and over a period of time and will not concern us at the doses we are considering, especially with the *all important* self-monitoring.

For the sake of completeness, we should just run through overdose problems. First of all, it is obvious that symptoms of the over-active thyroid are going to occur: palpitations, weight loss, oversensitivity to heat, tremors, anxiety and so on. Over a longer period the rapid heart beat might prove damaging and precipitate heart failure; but this is only seen with neglected hyperthyroidism or severe or prolonged overdosage. With the self-monitoring that I encouraged among my patients, this just doesn't happen.

Another spectre of overdosage is osteoporosis. This occurs with thyroxine overdosage especially but *not* at the physiological levels we are discussing. There is in fact no convincing evidence in the literature of osteoporosis from thyroid treatment, but establishment medicine uses the threat of this shrilly to warn against management using patient monitoring where the blood tests don't seem to fit. Osteoporosis is a real risk where oestrogen and progesterone levels are allowed to drop without replacement. More of this anon.

Another loudly expressed contraindication is the so-called risk of heart disease. In fact the reverse is the case. There has to be caution exercised if the heart is already damaged or weakened by disease, or has an irregular beat. Thyroid replacement of any degree has to be properly thought out and cautious, since the stimulation of heart activity when the machinery is damaged may well exaggerate the damage.

In forty years as a doctor, you learn one thing beyond all doubt: human beings are all different. Some are nice, some are nasty. The chemistry of one may be unbelievably different from the chemistry of another; one may make a textbook response to a treatment, while in another, all sorts of problems and complications may startle the patient and confound the physician.

In the treatment of thyroid and adrenal insufficiency, where there are so many different threads weaving and interweaving, this is especially true. Overall there is the hypothalamus, responding to all that goes on in the outside world, the slings and arrows of outrageous fortune. Our hopes and fears and all the other stresses that make up our daily life. The hypothalamus is in overall charge of the whole show, trying to keep up with all the changes internal and external that go on all the time.

What I am saying is that your response to treatment may be uneven; there will be good days and bad days. For example, you may have had a (strong) conversation with your loved one just before you leave, clutching an extremely unpleasant brown envelope; then find that the boss wants to see you as soon as you get into work. However many pills you take, you are going to have a bad couple of days. Sometimes you may find yourself full of energy and determination; sometimes you might feel quite the opposite. And the longer you have been ill, the longer and more difficult may be your recovery. This applies especially to people where low adrenal reserve has been a particular problem. But I can assure you that recovery is within your grasp; your life will change for the better, even perhaps more than you had ever hoped for.

Life is never simple, and nowhere is this more evident than in the treatment of metabolic disorders. There are spin-offs affecting other systems in the body and we need now to explore where these fit in and how they can be dealt with.

Chapter Ten

The Full Treatment Protocol

Thyroid illness is the Great Pretender – most especially the under-active thyroid. It can show up as almost any other illness you care to name. There may be dozens of symptoms which are diagnosed as a different illness, get treated on their merits, with the main, and underlying cause not thought about.

But in the same way the under-active thyroid may bring with it other problems related to it, even partly caused by it, and these need to be thought about whenever hypothyroidism is diagnosed. If these related problems are not considered, then the thyroid treatment may be unsatisfactory, or not work at all.

So we have a check list, or protocol, which has to be gone through when the original assessment is made of what may appear a straightforward hypothyroid state.

This is the list.

1.   ***Thyroid function:***   production of hormone

                                  transport of hormone

                                  conversion (T4 → T3)

                                  tissue receptor uptake

2.   ***Adrenal function:***   low adrenal reserve

                                  cortisol/DHEA imbalance

3.   ***Sex hormones:***   imbalance

                                  perimenopausal or menopausal insufficiency

4.   ***Presence of:***   systemic candida

                                  resulting in: leaky gut and gut dysbiosis

5.   ***Food allergies and intolerances***

6.   ***Malabsorption***

7.   ***Poor detoxification in the liver***

Problems with the **thyroid**, and with the **adrenals**, have their own chapters, which you will have got to grips with already. So now we have to think about the others.

Sex Hormones

I discussed these at length in Chapter Seven, so I will remind you of some of the basics only. This is more complicated for the ladies – no surprise there – because there is oestrogen and progesterone to work the whole thing. Men have, of course, testosterone.

Proper production of progesterone is pretty essential for successful implantation of the ovum, and this production is very sensitive to the right amount of thyroid hormone. If this is low, the progesterone is low. This will mean implantation either won't occur at all, or fouls up later on, with miscarriage. Oestrogen without progesterone to balance it, allows oestrogen dominance to occur, causing bloating, mood swings, in fact PMT, which may be really very severe. So low thyroid function is associated with PMT and infertility.

Since all hormones are related to each other, each requiring good activity of the others to work properly, low oestrogen and low progesterone affect thyroid production and take up; consequently, it may well be a good thing to consider some level of hormone replacement. *Not*, I hasten to say, the synthetic pills and patches, which are now under a cloud because of a renewed risk of promoting cancer, especially of the breast, but in a natural form, available as a cream. Progesterone and a mix of the three oestrogens are readily available, and provided you carefully follow the directions, are effective and safe.

It's worth mentioning in passing, that the failing production of oestrogen, progesterone and testosterone can be taken over, to a substantial degree, by healthy adrenal glands. Progesterone is formed from pregnenolone, and oestrogen and testosterone from DHEA. (Have a look at the adrenal cascade (Figure 10, Chapter Seven) again to see how this is done.) If the adrenals are showing signs of wear and tear, these hormones are going to be too low, so that low adrenal reserve is likely to mean a menopause worse than it need be.

One of the hazards of reduction of the sex hormones in both sexes is the loss of calcium from the bones. Low progesterone in the ladies may be associated with osteoporosis developing as early as their forties; low oestrogen also, although progesterone is more effective in treating it. Testosterone helps to grow new tissues, muscles and bones, and hence is especially important in men, who, without enough of it, can get osteoporosis as well. But it can also be used, with obvious care, in women.

To summarise then, estimating the current status of the sex hormones has to be part of the checking out and treatment of thyroid and adrenal problems. Before mid-life, imbalances may be self-correcting if the thyroid deficiency is corrected, and no intervention may be needed; but after mid-life some intervention is much more likely to be required, and forms an essential part of the overall treatment.

Candida

It's really only over recent decades that the full significance of **candida albicans**, the worst of the varieties, and probably the commonest, has been appreciated. It used to be thought that it was limited to small children whose bottles weren't properly sterilised, or to women, or was merely a cause of rashes or nail infections.

But candida is an endemic, silent destroyer, because wherever the immune system is compromised, candida will rear its ugly head. Candida is a fungus, which has a relatively innocuous resting state, and a really nasty active state, where it bores its way into and through tissues in order to reproduce its evil self. When it does this, you get all the usual expected symptoms; but if it has taken over the intestines, or indeed other tissues, it can cause all sorts of ongoing problems. Boring its way through the lining of the small intestine it opens channels, causing only partly digested foodstuffs to enter the circulation, which in their partly digested state, stimulate allergic response of the immune system. This is horribly inconvenient, since as time goes on, you become allergic to all sorts of different foods which previously had no effect.

Moreover, candida has another sinister role to play. It is normally kept in check by beneficial bacteria in the small intestine: the good guys. These include lactobacillus, bacteroides and bifidobacteria, which, in addition to keeping our insides healthy, have a part to play in the integrity of our immune system. The presence of candida, and the toxins it produces, has the effect of edging out these good guys, and replacing them with the mob. These include klebsiella, pseudomonas, and clostridia; when this happens it is called dysbiosis.

Dysbiosis is bad news since it inevitably means that intestinal health is damaged and the overall immune system compromised. In addition, this situation promotes 'leaky gut'. The **leaky gut** syndrome means (i) antigens passing into the bloodstream, (ii) pathogens also entering the bloodstream, (iii) toxins similarly and (iv) undigested food in the blood.

We are likely, as a result, to suffer from inflammatory, autoimmune and allergic diseases. Probably the most common presentation of this is the irritable bowel syndrome (IBS) in its various guises, and it is possible that Crohn's disease may have its original cause in this process. The entrance of toxins means an overload situation on a liver already in trouble from low metabolism.

Candida has a lot to answer for and we should do all we can to eliminate it as far as possible; however good the treatment of the thyroid and adrenal problems, candida will prevent proper response and recovery.

Its treatment falls into four sections. First, you try to starve it out. Candida thrives on sugar – so much so, it can actually make you crave sugar and starch. It's impossible to eliminate carbohydrates completely, but you can cut out all refined sugars and starches, and have high fibre fruit and vegetables – the complex carbohydrates.

Second, we must try to kill the candida with fungicide. Nystatin has long been popular; another is Sporonox. I recommend, partly for the sake of simplicity, Fluconazole (without prescription), 1 x 150 mg weekly, for 2 or 3 weeks, which can be very effective; more so if combined with caprylic acid or grapefruit seed extract, garlic or horopito. Essential is the provision of the beneficial bacteria to replace the mob; these are the pre- and probiotics which contain millions of the beneficial bacteria and the food to feed them. All health food shops can recommend effective preparations.

You have to go on with the treatment for weeks or even months; the good news is that as your metabolism comes back to normal it will control re-infection, an ever present risk. (Worsened by antibiotics, the pill and phyto-oestrogens.) You may have several days of feeling really awful when there is a massive candida die off. Don't worry; it will pass and proves that the need was great.

To test for candida there is the old-fashioned test often used by nutritionists where you have a good spit into a glass of water on waking. If your spit starts to form tails and looks like a small jellyfish there is a good chance that candida is present. To confirm this you can do a salivary antibody test, which is a most reliable way of making the diagnosis. These tests are available from private laboratories (see Appendix D).

Food Allergies and Intolerances

Most of us are familiar with gluten/wheat allergy – indeed, many of us have allergies to wheat; but almost as common are allergies to milk, eggs, citrus fruits, shellfish, the potato family (which includes tomatoes and peppers), together with intolerances to certain chemicals and additives. The difficulty with these allergies is that since they occur in common foodstuffs, we may not be aware of them as a cause of our symptoms. These symptoms may include chronic stomach upsets, skin problems, sinus catarrh, asthma, headaches, fatigue, anxiety and depression. The allergic response is masked by the exposure to the allergen on a daily basis, which commonly relieves the worst of the symptoms, rather like withdrawal from a drug; as soon as you have your 'fix' the symptoms largely disappear.

There are various ways of spotting these ongoing problems. The Vega machine is very popular, kinesiology can pick many up, and the Rast blood test may also be helpful. Probably the most sure way to check them out is an exclusion diet. For about ten days you have absolutely no contact with the suspect food. During this time, after two or three days the allergic response is 'unmasked', and the symptoms it is causing become more obvious. You come out in a rash, get a crashing headache, suffer from an unreasonable depression, and then in a few more days all the symptoms go and you feel really better. This can be followed by a 'challenge test': for wheat, as an example, you gnaw a fine hunk of bread. If you feel terrible after a few hours – not immediately, and it may take a day – then you have learnt something. Most people do actually have dark suspicions about certain foodstuffs upsetting them and are already being careful. If you are not sure, you really might like to check it out – especially gluten, which can actually block thyroid hormone production.

Malabsorption

Many people have a tendency to digest their food less well as the years pass by – one reason why some people lose weight even if they are apparently eating quite well. This is more likely if the metabolism is below normal. As I have said elsewhere, nothing works properly, including digestion. You stop producing stomach acid normally (this is called **hypochlorhydria**) and the digestive enzymes from the pancreas run down as well. The effect is to have digestive upsets, often indigestion, which can get put down to too much acid and treated with antacids, which of course makes the whole thing worse. If levels of vitamins and minerals are checked, they are often low across the board. This obviously means that you have malnutrition to cope with as well as your low metabolism, which is going to worsen the whole picture greatly. Weight loss and bowel upsets should put you on your guard. If you need to establish the possibility, a **combined digestive and stool analysis (CDSA)** will soon point to the problem.

The treatment is to have the acid and enzymes replaced. For the stomach, betaine hydrochloride is used before meals. For the pancreas there are a number of enzymes available from health food shops. I often recommend Nutrigest from Nutri Ltd, which combines both.

Liver Detoxification

The liver is amazing. Something like 2 quarts of blood is filtered every minute to enable it to deal with every possible toxin that our environment, and even our own metabolic processes, can throw at us. Many of these chemicals it neutralises in different ways, changes them and then gets rid of them, through the bile or the kidneys via the bloodstream. If we bombard our long-suffering livers with chemicals of various sorts – benzpyrenes, alcohol, caffeine, food additives – we can obviously overstretch the liver resources and suffer from our indulgence. But if our metabolism is running down, the complex machinery starts to suffer and the liver cannot do its job properly and begins to suffer from toxicity.

One approach must be to bring our metabolism on line so that the liver can actually work properly. But we can also approach it from the other direction, and by detoxifying the overloaded liver help speed up the process of regaining our metabolic health. To start with, we stay away from saturated fats, refined sugars and alcohol.

Foods that help promote healthy liver function are: (i) high sulphur foods, such as garlic, legumes, onions, and eggs; (ii) water soluble fibre, such as pears, oatbran, apples, and legumes; (iii) cabbage family vegetables (cook them properly!); (iv) artichokes, beets, carrots, tumeric, cinnamon, and legumes. The herb milk thistle (silymarin) is very good for cleansing the liver. You also need nutrient supplements – a high dose multivitamin and mineral preparation; vitamin C, betacarotene and vitamin E are a must.

For detoxification, fasting has long been used – a week long fast can dramatically improve the overall health of the liver. Better, perhaps, than outright starvation, is the use of fresh fruit and vegetable juices two or three days a week for a month or so. You have three or four 8-12 oz juice meals over the day, together with the high potency vitamins and minerals, a significant amount of vitamin C – say 3 grams – fibre supplements and silymarin, say 70 to 200 mg, 3 times a day. In general, rest is pretty important (so it is best done at the weekend); plenty of pure water and light exercise only (that is your walk to the local shops and back). An almost immediate improvement in well-being can be expected, and a liver detox should come high on the agenda in regaining our metabolic health.

Chapter Eleven

Reverse T3
and Wilson's Syndrome

I have already touched on reverse T3 (rT3) and some of you reading this book may well have already come across it, looking through information leaflets, or in snippets from booklets or perhaps on the net, and wondered perhaps, how it related to you. Well, let's find out.

You won't need reminding by now about the whys and wherefores of T3; just the same, that is what I am going to do. You remember the molecule of T4 drawn in Chapter Two with its four iodine atoms (Figure 4). We pictured it as two rings linked together by an oxygen atom (in fact, these are better pictured in three dimensions as one ring situated over the other) and to each of these rings iodine atoms are attached. Under the action of the 5'-deiodinase enzymes, one of the iodine atoms from the outer ring is removed; this is called deiodination and we are left with T3, which you remember does all the work.

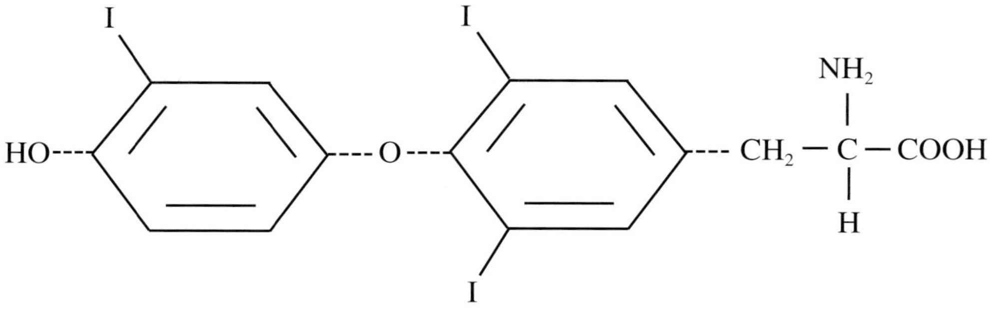

Figure 13. (T3) 3,5,3'-tri-iodothyronine (liothyronine)

However, it is also possible to remove an iodine atom from the inner ring; the molecule is almost the same, but not quite, and the end result is an 'isomer' of T3, called, to give it its full chemical name 3,3',5'-tri-iodothyronine (rT3). You will recall that isomers are compounds which are chemically the same, with the same number of atoms and everything, *but arranged differently.*

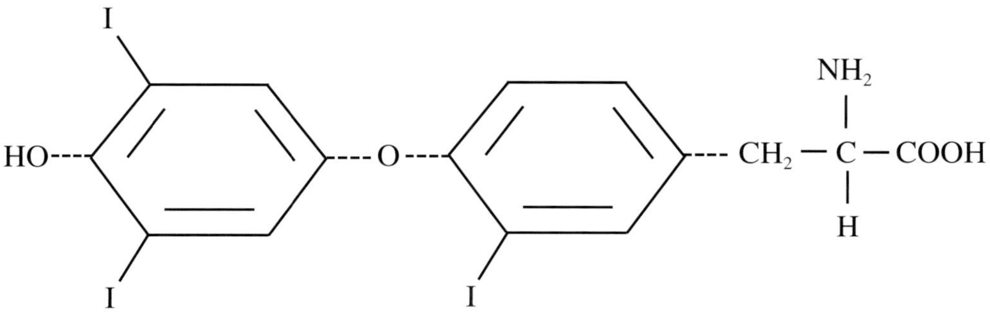

Figure 14. (rT3) 3,3',5'-tri-iodothyronine

rT3 was first recognised in 1956, and was quickly found to be a product of thyroid metabolism actually within the cell. The thyroid itself makes very little indeed – about 5% in all – between 1.2 and 4.2 mcg a day – so that nearly all of it is made in the tissues by the deiodination process of T4, and in the normal run of things there isn't much to be found anyway: something like 40 micrograms per day all told in the bloodstream. Its activity in affecting metabolism is virtually nil; it is about 5% of the power of T4, which has very little effect anyway.

Since it apparently does not do anything, you may well ask what is it for? Well, it is extremely useful for recycling iodine, and it disappears much more rapidly than T3 – which is fast enough – as the body breaks it down to release the iodine. But its main function is to lower the amount of active, normal T3 in the system when it is surplus to requirements.

Basically, this happens in various non-thyroidal disease states. In thyroid illness, it works much as you would expect; it is low in hypothyroidism, and high in hyperthyroidism. However, it occasionally happens that the mechanism goes out of kilter and the body manufactures much more rT3 than it should. In this situation there will be a greater or lesser degree of hypothyroidism, since a proportion of the T3 is unusable. This is the stand taken by Dr Denis Wilson of which more in a moment. T3 becomes lower in starvation and other debilitating illnesses; and in the obese patient undergoing a fast, the T3 goes down and the rT3 goes up. These same changes occur in cirrhosis of the liver and insulin dependent diabetes mellitus (IDDM), and surgery causes a rise in rT3 within 24 hours.

A special case concerns the baby *in utero*; it produces much of its thyroid hormones as rT3 until birth. If the mother, however, is actually hypothyroid, she borrows some of the baby's thyroid in the normal form. This has two results: the mother may be fine during her pregnancy, but goes down with a bang afterwards and the thyroid hormone acts as a growth hormone in the baby, with the result that the baby may be extra heavy. This as we noted earlier is one of the two chief causes of overweight babies, the other being diabetes mellitus.

Wilson's syndrome

In 1991 Dr Wilson in the USA described a variation of thyroid illness to which he attached his name. Many physicians are not convinced by any means that it is in fact a distinct syndrome, nor, not to put too fine a point on it, that it justifies an eponymous title. Be that as it may.

He hypothesized a sustained **euthyroid sick syndrome**. He asserted that the problem lay in a partial failure of the conversion of T4 to T3. He defined the condition as 'The cluster of often debilitating symptoms especially brought on by significant physical or emotional states, that can persist even after the stress has passed, which responds characteristically to the special thyroid treatment...' (That he advocates.) He says it is typified by a body temperature running on average below normal, with routine blood tests often in the normal range. He went on to say that it is 'A survival mechanism that has gotten stuck', and thatit results in 'multiple enzyme dysfunction caused by variations in body temperature'.

There appears to be no reliable evidence to support his stuck survival mechanism theory but no-one would disagree with his other symptoms and signs; after all, they are no different from what we have been learning about already.

What he says happens is that as a result of dieting and/or stress the body makes too much rT3 at the expense of T3 itself; and this mechanism remains 'stuck' afterwards. Other authorities dispute this, saying that after dieting or stress everything reverts to normal within one or two weeks anyway. He summarises his position as follows: (i) During fasting there is a decrease of T3. (ii) Fasting thus slows down the metabolic rate. (iii) This state may persist.

It has to be said that there really is little evidence to support Dr Wilson's contention, although as we know, illness and life events may cause permanent thyroid damage, but whether because of the rT3/T3 problem is really not clear. My own view is that there is poor T4 → T3 conversion and low T3 uptake by tissue receptors as a result of receptor resistance, together with a failure to produce sufficient DHEA and cortisol.

Dr Wilson's treatment consists of managing the patient on high and increasing doses of T3 (usually in a specially prepared sustained release form) broken up by episodes without treatment. This, he claims, brings the natural mechanism back on line.

My problem (as with many others) is that high doses of T3 *ab initio* may cause a number of hyperthyroid side effects, which may be most uncomfortable if not actually dangerous. Also, many patients with poor conversion will respond to T3 anyway, but the doses do not need to be so high. In summary, I, along with others, am far from convinced that his approach brings any useful advantages in the treatment of hypothyroidism. T3 has a most important part to play where there are conversion problems and should, additionally, be used to balance the use of T4 in any but the mildest degree of hypothyroidism.

Chapter Twelve

The Parathyroid Glands

As you will have understood by now, the thyroid affects not only all the tissues and organs of the body but also the other hormones; in turn, the healthy activity of the thyroid can be affected by these hormones. It is clear that we must understand how they all fit in and what their roles are, so we are now going to examine the role of the parathyroid glands.

Many people are a bit unclear in their minds about the parathyroid glands, since the name suggests that there ought to be a connection with the thyroid itself and its metabolic hormones. I may as well say at the outset that, actually, apart from being positioned very close to the thyroid, they really have no connection with the running of the metabolism. They do, however, have a relationship with the thyroid when it comes to the control of calcium.

There are four parathyroid glands, which are paired. Two just above the thyroid and two just below. Rarely, they are out of position as a result of developmental anomalies, but usually this does not interfere with their function. They are very small, only a few millimetres across and are mustard yellow in colour. They were first described in 1925 and medical students were always taught to associate them with Moans, Groans and Stones. Their job in life (together with calcitonin in the thyroid) is to control the calcium level of the bloodstream within quite a narrow range, something like between 2.25 and 2.65 mmol/L, or 9 to 10.4 mg/100 ml. Figure 15, opposite, explains how it all works.

Calcium plays a crucial role in the correct function of nerve stimuli, most especially at the interface between nerve and muscle. The parathyroid glands work this control by secreting the parathyroid hormone (PTH) into the bloodstream when the blood levels of calcium are low, and calcitonin is secreted from the thyroid when the blood levels are high. So when PTH is released, this has the effect of allowing the osteoclast cells in the bones to release some of the calcium they hold, thus increasing calcium blood levels. PTH also affects intestinal absorption of calcium and an increase will allow more calcium to pass from the digestive tract into the bloodstream.

Calcitonin is made by certain thyroid cells, the parafollicular cells, and acts to lower circulating levels of calcium (as you see in the diagram) working against the parathyroid hormone. Vitamin D, metabolised to 1,25-dihydroxyvitamin D_3, also has a part to play, increasing serum calcium levels.

Parathyroid activity has no link with thyroid hormone production, although it may be influenced by the thyroid stimulating hormone (TSH). A poorly functioning thyroid cannot produce calcitonin adequately, but, oddly enough, this doesn't seem to matter very much; the parathyroid glands appear to be able to undertake the regulation of calcium levels by themselves.

The mechanism can go wrong in two ways: producing too much PTH or producing too little. Producing too much, hyperparathyroidism, is in general the result of a

Figure 15. Calcium balance

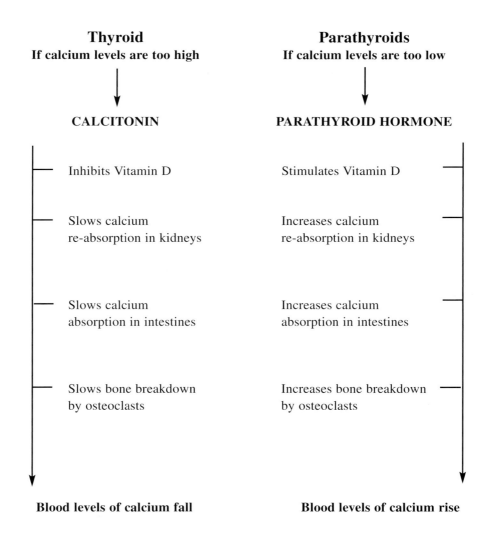

Thyroid **If calcium levels are too high**	**Parathyroids** **If calcium levels are too low**
CALCITONIN	**PARATHYROID HORMONE**
Inhibits Vitamin D	Stimulates Vitamin D
Slows calcium re-absorption in kidneys	Increases calcium re-absorption in kidneys
Slows calcium absorption in intestines	Increases calcium absorption in intestines
Slows bone breakdown by osteoclasts	Increases bone breakdown by osteoclasts
Blood levels of calcium fall	**Blood levels of calcium rise**

hormone-producing tumour – a parathyroid adenoma – which usually affects just one of the four parathyroids in about 90% of cases. Rarely, they may all enlarge – 'parathyroid hyperplasia' – for reasons not especially understood. Should biochemistry of the blood reveal excess calcium, a special scan is undertaken at hospital. This Sestambi scan relies on a protein labelled with a radioactive isotope, Technetium-99, which is taken up by the demands of the over-active parathyroid gland, and when scanned, of course, shows up as a hot spot. The other normal parathyroids go into a dormant state and show no activity.

Too much calcium in the blood has a number of effects. Not least, of course, is the loss of calcium in the bones, which will weaken them by osteoporosis. Most people feel generally unwell, with poor sleep, irritability and some memory loss (moans). Also noticed is an increased tendency to gastric ulceration and pancreatitis (groans) and the classic problem is the production of kidney stones as a result of the high levels of calcium passing through them (stones). Bones breaking with unusual ease (pathological fractures) are another sign of this. Treatment of hyperparathyroidism lies in removing the over-active parathyroid, which will provide a complete cure.

Low calcium, as with hypoparathyroidism, affects the nervous and muscular system and may be the result of the parathyroid glands being affected by autoimmune attack in the same way as the thyroid and adrenal glands. There is general weakness, poor blood pressure control, and a tendency to tingling in the hands and feet and possible heart irregularities. There may be spasms or partial paralysis. (This can be brought on, on purpose, by hyperventilation or over-breathing, when the loss of carbon dioxide has the effect of reducing available calcium.) The extreme case is the *main d'accoucheur*, which is a paralysis of the hands picturesquely described as the hand of an obstetrician while delivering the baby. Eventually, unconsciousness supervenes. This 'calcium tetany' may be seen not uncommonly in the elderly and there is an increased risk of osteoporosis. The loss of calcium in hypoparathyroidism may be relieved by an injection of the calcium salt followed by regular calcium supplements.

Generally speaking, the condition is relatively uncommon and unlikely to be a problem with thyroid disease. It has happened though, that since the parathyroids are so small, they have come out by mistake during thyroidectomy. If all four do, calcium tetany will follow – quickly relieved, however, by an injection of calcium. However, none of this should interfere with the diagnosis or treatment of thyroid and adrenal function but should be one of the simple checks made when blood chemistry is undertaken.

Finally, I would like to mention an unusual condition called pseudo-hypoparathyroidism. This is a genetically inherited condition in which the patients have obesity, round face, short stature, shortening of the bones in the hands and a tendency to produce nodules of calcium here and there in the body. These patients turn out to have too much phosphate and too little calcium in the bloodstream as if they weren't producing enough parathyroid hormone. In fact, they are. What happens, however, is that the receptor sites are unable to respond properly to the parathyroid hormone and therefore a situation arises as if there was too little. This failure is the result of an inability of another of the G proteins in the receptor sites to respond as they should, and this deficiency may cause a failure of response to other hormones including the thyroid hormones. So this is a rare instance where hypothyroidism may have a connection with the parathyroids.

Chapter Thirteen

Chronic Fatigue and the Thyroid Factor

Studies over the past few years have cast a bright light in the darkness and confusion surrounding this illness. It has several names, which all mean very much the same thing. **Myalgic encephalomyelitis (ME)** and **chronic fatigue syndrome (CFS)** are those by which it is most known in the United Kingdom. **Post viral fatigue (PVF)** is another one and in the USA it is best known as **fibromyalgia**. It began as the 'The Royal Free disease' (the actual cause at the time was a virus causing Bornholm's disease), and has laboured under the nickname 'yuppie flu'. I am going to use the term chronic fatigue syndrome (CFS) for the sake of clarity.

Even today many physicians and consultants won't admit to its existence, mostly because (i) the patient isn't to be believed and is making the whole thing up, and (ii) standard blood tests show nothing wrong anyway. Patients get a pretty hard time from such doctors, who, if they don't diagnose simple lead swinging (they write *plumborum pendularum* on their certificates), will put their patients on a variety of antidepressants. Those doctors who do listen to their patients may nevertheless find that they are more or less powerless to help very much.

For myself, I have been treating CFS for many years, based on the fact that the underlying problem is a down-regulation of their metabolic status, a definition for which we have to thank Dr John Lowe, who has done more to help patients than any other doctor in this field. Broadly speaking, this means that adrenal and thyroid insufficiency are at the root of many of the presenting symptoms.

I have found patients fall into four categories. There is one group, about half of all who seek advice, and who most importantly have not been ill for very long. These patients tend to get better within weeks or months and can expect to recover their health completely. About one quarter of the rest make some improvement and may be able to live relatively normal lives but no matter what one does, return to full health eludes them. Of the remaining quarter, half really don't get better at all and the physicians and the patients alike remain disappointed, and the other half not only show no improvement at all; but indeed seem if anything to get worse and become thoroughly disenchanted with any treatment offered. They have been ill for so long that they can no longer believe that there is ever any chance of getting well and may even become emotionally attached to their lifestyle. There are of course some patients who confound everybody and get better, as I am fond of saying, *in spite* of treatment. For these the illness runs its course, maybe for a year or more, and their immune system finally defeats it. But it may well mean a long time out of someone's life; especially as it tends to attack younger people, notably teenagers with all the disaster that inevitably is brought to their lives and careers.

The main problem, of course, is that no-one really agrees quite what CFS is and anyway, the illness has different facets and there can be no doubt that different aspects may be emphasised from patient to patient. However, we can certainly explain how it starts, the way it affects people, and its variable course.

Most commonly it begins with a viral illness; a major operation, or major life event also come quite high on the list. Glandular fever must be about the most common factor, bad influenza nearly as common and then there may be other illnesses from which recovery never seems complete. The glandular fever or influenza doesn't seem to run a normal course; the usual recovery just doesn't happen and the patient remains exhausted and ill after minor exertion, suffering from symptoms which get better and relapse again. If we consider glandular fever as a good example, the whole thing starts with a sore throat and fever. After a few days the illness persists and the doctor may be persuaded to give antibiotics. Usually they make no difference. A throat swab grows none of the usual organisms that cause sore throats – and the sore throat and fever persist. Blood tests may provide a clue. The monocyte count (one of the groups of white blood cells) may be raised – hence the other name for the illness: infectious mononucleosis – and if tests are done for the virus causing the infection, the Epstein Barr, Coxsackie, or cytomegalovirus *may* show up.

Unfortunately, none of this gets us anywhere because glandular fever is virtually impossible to treat. And there may be a problem with the immune system in the first place, compromised by unsuspected deficiencies. And to understand how this could be, we need to understand a little about the essential fatty acids. There are three groups which we obtain from our diet. The omega-3, omega-6, and omega-9 group. Under the action of enzymes these form families essential for many life processes, in particular to form and maintain healthy cell membranes necessary for cells to communicate with each other and the body as a whole. The omega-3 and omega-6 families produce derivatives called eicosanoids, which play crucial roles in controlling inflammation, blood clotting and healing processes.

It's the omega-3 family that concerns us because of the alpha-linolenic acid that heads it, and is the commonest omega-3 to be found in contemporary diets, is turned by an enzyme (delta-6-desaturase) into another very important fatty acid called eicosapentaenoic acid (EPA). This kills viruses, and produces under the action of other enzymes (cyclo-oxygenase and lipo-oxygenase), powerful immune chemicals called interferons. So EPA kills off foreign viral invaders.

All very well you might say, so why don't they work sometimes? It turns out that some viruses can inactivate the delta-6-desaturase enzyme making the EPA and so it doesn't get made properly, and can't kill off the viruses.

We are all chronically short of omega-3 essential fatty acids because of deficiencies and toxins in our diet; and some of us, all unknowing, therefore cannot fight off certain viral infections. Large doses of vitamin C have been recommended in some quarters; I have found that a short sharp dose of a corticosteroid may short circuit the illness. But in general, the patient has to rest and let time and healing take their course. Hopefully, most will throw the illness off in two or three weeks. But, sadly, some don't. Symptoms remain, coming and going, with no apparent end. Life now becomes beset with episodes of fever, sore throat, complete exhaustion, stomach upsets, aching and stiffness in the joints, poor sleep, headaches and a constant feeling of malaise. Other symptoms include night sweats, depression, visual disturbances, cognitive dysfunction and motion sickness. As this goes on advice is sooner or later sought. Usually nothing turns up, and the patient is told to rest, and rest, and rest and be patient. At this point someone will be saying CFS, ME, fibromyalgia. This means that no recovery can be expected within a certain, and perhaps long, time and the patient has to alter their whole lifestyle, even to being an invalid for an indefinite time.

Most patients become more or less unable to work, and have to draw sickness benefit. The problem can sometimes be that the opting out of society may, to some people, be rather a relief, which may delay their recovery or at least their perception of recovery. One thing one always learns in medicine is that everyone responds to their illness in a different way. Someone with a broken leg may remain in a wheel chair or on crutches for weeks; others, eyes alight with determination, will be lurching about unaided within a week or so. The same applies to CFS.

Going through the literature one is struck by the enormous amount that has been written on the subject of CFS. Like many things in life, the amount written is often in inverse proportion to what is actually known, and especially what can actually be done to make people better. CFS is probably the best example ever. There are great exceptions in the extraordinary and deep research carried out by Dr John Lowe, Dr Joseph Teitelbaum and Dr Goldstein in the USA, who have made sense of all that is actually known. I shall be drawing heavily in this chapter on their work and have been constantly sustained by the parallels in thinking that we share.

We agree in pointing out straight away, that there is a constant tussle between the proponents of some form of rheumatoid illness and those who believe the whole thing is basically psychosomatic. The lone voices who point to adrenal and thyroid dysfunction and consequent down-regulation of metabolism as a major cause are ridiculed and vilified by the establishment in the USA, as they are indeed in the United Kingdom. Partly, one regrets to say, the poor general understanding of thyroid disorders plays a major role in this. In the USA there is a powerful lobby that considers the condition to be entirely due to hysteria and psychiatric problems, and this is now establishment standard thinking in the UK; and the psychiatrists have very strong vested interests.

While it is clear that hypothyroidism with all its obvious symptoms and signs should be evident to patient and doctor alike, there are one or two other aspects of thyroid dysfunction which I must talk about. One is **euthyroid hypometabolism** (and I am drawing a distinction here from the sick euthryoid syndrome) and the other is **thyroid hormone resistance**.

Euthyroid hypometabolism is low cellular metabolism despite normal thyroid function tests. The tissues simply are unable to respond properly to the thyroid hormones. This occurs, for example, notably with low adrenal function. This may occur where the feedback loop governing ACTH secretion from the pituitary (to increase adrenal function) doesn't work properly. It should be clear that simply increasing thyroid hormone (thyroxine) from outside may well not work; the tissues are unable to respond. Many of these patients may respond to liothyronine, T3, provided the adrenal status is also considered as part of the treatment. At a small risk of belabouring the point we can conveniently list some four causes of failure to diagnose euthyroid hypometabolism:

1. Psychoneurosis is the preferred diagnosis. Encouraged by vested interests but a false concept.

2. CFS. 'It is very rare so it doesn't really happen.'

3. Hypothyroidism. It may, indeed, be hidden hypothyroidism, but is not considered bad enough to treat.

4. Uptake failure. There is no evidence that the thyroid hormones fail to act where they should. (There is ample, of course.)

To place this in perspective, I want to highlight for a moment the work of Dr John Lowe in the USA, who has written a treatise, probably the most complete available, on *The Metabolic Treatment of Fibromyalgia* (see Appendix D) and he has conducted a number of trials and written a number of papers on this basis. The majority of his patients he found had degrees of thyroid malfunction, in particular an inability to convert T4 → T3. His conclusions are I believe unassailable.

1. Fibromyalgia is a syndrome of signs and symptoms resulting from hypometabolism.

2. In most cases the hypometabolism has multiple causes.

3. The usual presentation is of poor thyroid hormone regulation due to either hypothyroidism, conversion block or partial cellular resistance. These features are complicated and made worse by low adrenal reserve and poor nutrition, sex hormone imbalances and poor physical fitness.

4. 85% recover from illness by treating the hypometabolism and the T3 route will always be much superior to the use of T4.

The paper published in the *Journal of Chronic Fatigue Syndrome*, by Dr Jacob Teiltelbaum and colleagues in 2001, pointed out that the syndrome is a multifactorial illness with various symptoms noted in varying degrees, so that treatment has to be tailored to the patient. He and his colleagues undertook a most thoughtful and careful study on the response to treatment on these lines.

Most patients received some kind of night sedation of a simple and non-addictive kind, and some received low dosage antidepressants. Most were provided with nutritional support with iron, vitamin C and other vitamins including B_{12} injections. Thyroid, either Armour thyroid or synthetic thyroid hormone, T4 or T3, was given to more than half of the patients with obvious thyroid symptoms and/or positive blood tests. Cortisone and DHEA were given to more than half of the patients in the trial. Some men were given testosterone and some women oestrogen, where shown to be deficient. High levels of fungus in the stools was treated with nystatin and abnormal bacteria concentrations in the stool (e.g. *Closteridium difficile*) was treated with metronidazole.

The result of the study was quite unequivocal. They were gratified to find in this trial that 48.5% of patients were much better and 42% were somewhat better; an extraordinarily encouraging result. It was concluded that the multifactorial problems of CFS should all receive attention, but that thyroid and adrenal support was a major factor.

While blood tests may be useful, it seems that chronic fatigue patients can manage themselves even if medical advice is unsympathetic. Natural thyroid and adrenal support as outlined in the chapter on self-help would seem pretty mandatory. You must sleep properly and fully; there are over-the-counter preparations or your doctor may be persuaded to help.

The use of thyroid and adrenal support for this condition is violently opposed by establishment physicians, and a number of skeletons in the cupboard are rattled sufficiently to convince patients and doctors not to dare to undertake trials of treatment. This treatment of course means natural thyroid and liothyronine, and the use of adrenal supplementation.

Thyroid hormone resistance or failure of thyroid hormone regulation can occur at several levels and is likely to be partial in degree. Broadly, the problem is that the tissues simply don't respond properly to the thyroid hormone, even though blood tests indicate that there is enough. It is worth making the point that tissues degraded by hypothyroidism are likely to respond poorly in any case, and any attempt to improve the blood levels is likely to cause overdose symptoms.

We can recognise three forms of thyroid hormone resistance: general, pituitary and peripheral. Without going into too much detail, the resistance occurs in:

1. The pituitary gland only, which does not respond to hypothalamic control hormones and the circulating blood levels of thyroid hormone.

2. The pituitary gland itself and target tissues.

3. Peripheral tissue resistance only.

We must mention again the Gq/11 connection; the G proteins switch on or switch off the activity of T3 in the cell and the manufacture of TSH. The Gq/11 connection, which switches off T3 response and TSH production, is sensitive to certain tissue poisons, most particularly fluorides, which cause it to overact in shutting down metabolism.

We can now see more clearly how the thyroid-adrenal axis, each function affecting the other, can cause the condition of lowered metabolic activity at all levels, which results in the syndrome we know as CFS/fibromyalgia/ME. No body tissue, no organ, no function escapes. But because we are so complex and no human being is quite like another, it may manifest itself in an infinite number of ways in detail, yet with the common overall picture of fatigue, depression, arthralgic pains, digestive problems and so on, that we have become familiar with. The government, that is establishment experts, are coming heavily down on the side of CFS as being fundamentally a psychiatric illness, in defiance of a vast body of evidence to the contrary, all available but not suitable for establishment eyes. Thousands of human beings are now labelled as *psychosomatic freaks* and condemned to a lifetime of chronic ill health and invalidism. Their treatment? Antidepressants, cognitive therapy, paced exercise and eventually they will get better. But they don't, which is of course their fault.

The conclusion is inescapable. CFS is an illness of deficiencies and thyroid dysfunction, and must be thought of in these terms with the treatment based on the correction of these deficiencies. As we have seen, thyroid and adrenal support is of crucial importance, and there are multiple nutritional and other considerations which can be corrected and dealt with.

And now we must deal with the essential fatty acid deficiencies. The approach is to provide enough of the eicosapentaenoic acid (EPA) so that the damaging effects of the chronic viral infection on the delta-6-saturase enzyme don't matter. Professor Basant Puri's work has shown that the use of very pure eicosapentaenoic acid, together with high quality gamma-linoleic oil (which belongs to the omega-6 family) from evening primrose oil has shown most encouraging results. He recommends a product of especial quality called VegEPA (see Appendix D). This targets the viral load, which, from severe flu or glandular fever most commonly, may have started the whole thing off. His results from the use of these supplements have been very encouraging, and consideration should certainly be given to a broad approach encompassing this treatment and the treatment of metabolic deficiency as well.

To summarise. In ME/CFS/fibromyalgia, thyroid and adrenal deficiencies must be identified and treated, using natural products and nutrients where possible. Other glandular deficiencies must also be treated. Candida must be ruthlessly dealt with and the damage corrected by using probiotics and prebiotics (the good bacteria and its required food). Malabsorption must be corrected. There should be active replacement of eicosapentaenoic acid (EPA) together with gamma-linoleic acid (GLA).

The successful approach to ME/CFS/fibromyalgia has to be on several fronts. A natural, non-drug approach is infinitely better than the heavy and desperate use of antidepressants. We have to remember that many of you have been ill for years and that the healing that occurs may take time as the system repairs and learns again how to work.

Although you may feel that what I have said, along with the other committed researchers I have mentioned, is really pretty reasonable, it is fashionable in the UK at least, to regard it all as really rather fringe stuff, and certainly not establishment doctrine. But studies *do* show that CFS is a multifactorial illness with very definite physical changes in the nervous systems and body chemistry, and treatment has to be individualised and customised for each and every patient. The most recent paper by Dr Teitelbaum and others showed beyond doubt the correctness of this approach and that his general philosophy of this illness has to be on the right lines. Professor Basant Puri's work and Dr John Lowe's definitive research should not fail to convert the most convinced sceptic. Unbelievably their arguments – as indeed mine – have met with considerable hostility from the medical establishment.

What I feel must be done is to marshal all the facts, and those patients who become convinced of the hypothalamic-pituitary axis and the thyroid-adrenal axis as playing a prime role in their illness, seek advice from like thinking doctors, or help themselves in the manner I have outlined earlier. You must sleep properly and fully. Your diet should be organic and wholesome, free from additives that wreak havoc on immune systems. Extra omega-3 and omega-6, iron, and vitamins, especially 1 or 2 grams of vitamin C daily would seem essential. You may seek help if your depression is really pulling you down, or you can use St John's wort. Obtain hormone and DHEA levels from saliva, blood or urine tests and insist on replacement therapy that is as natural as possible. Have your stools examined for parasites and/or fungus and have any such infections treated. Live Blood Analysis is an exciting new technique for screening blood for a number of systemic conditions, as well as parasites etc (see Appendix D). Be patient; follow these regimes for as long as it takes. There is no way you can be harmed by these measures and you have every chance of great improvement or cure and having your life restored to you.

Chapter Fourteen

The Thyroid and Diabetes

When I use the word diabetes, I am actually referring to **diabetes mellitus**. The other sort of diabetes is diabetes insipidus. The two are not remotely connected and the insipidus form is nothing to do with sugar. Both, however, can make you extremely thirsty as well as extremely ill.

To try to be as helpful as possible I will quickly get diabetes insipidus out of the way. What happens here is that there is a specific failure of one of the control functions of the pituitary gland; to be precise, the posterior pituitary, which in addition to producing the hormone oxytocin, which plays a vital role in childbirth, produces vasopressin or the anti-diuretic hormone (ADH). This hormone targets the kidneys, which are made to reabsorb most of the fluid they filter off from the bloodstream. A degree of failure of the posterior pituitary to make ADH, means the kidneys do not do the reabsorption properly, so that they produce excessive amounts of fluid. This of course makes one pass huge amounts of urine (polyuria) and drink like a fish (polydipsia). The condition can be extraordinarily unpleasant and disabling, though happily the missing hormone is easily given in a snuff, breathed up two or three times a day. As a matter of interest, people with hypothyroidism of some severity and long-standing, and consequent imbalance of the pituitary-adrenal axis, do indeed have symptoms of excessive thirst and urination, especially at night.

Diabetes mellitus is very much more common and becoming more so. There are two kinds of diabetes mellitus, Type II non-insulin dependent diabetes (NIDD), which is the most common and also called late-onset mature diabetes, and Type I insulin dependent diabetes (IDD), which commonly follows a viral infection that destroys the insulin producing cells in the pancreas, the β cells in the islets of Langerhans.

In Type II diabetes, the insulin producing cells that control the level of sugar in the blood become less and less responsive to blood sugar levels, producing less insulin, and the receptors in the tissues become less able to respond to the insulin anyway. As a result the blood sugar level starts to rise, and the body becomes less able to tolerate carbohydrates – sugars and starches – and increasingly rids itself of the excess, loses it in the kidneys by the passage of excess water. So the diabetic is excessively thirsty and has to keep passing water. These patients tend to present as being overweight, tired, thirsty, with polyuria, itching and feeling generally unwell; they also have large babies. If the diabetes gets out of hand, as in Type I, weight loss can occur. This type of diabetes may be controlled by a low carbohydrate diet and/or drugs (eg the sulfonylureas), which improve output and absorption of the insulin. Untreated, the condition worsens until the patient lapses into coma and dies.

In Type I diabetes, the insulin producing cells don't do their job at all and the patient, who may be quite young, rapidly gets very ill with sudden weight loss, weakness, extreme thirst, polyuria, candida and itching. This condition cannot go untreated. These patients require their desperately needed insulin to be given by a regular injection to bring down their high sugar levels.

Other factors affect how much patients may be troubled by their diabetes mellitus. One is the element chromium, the addition of which to the diet can be quite vital. Environment has a major part to play, most especially excessive eating of the wrong foods and consequent obesity, which overrun your insulin producing capacity, and eventually exhaust the islet cells that produce it. Prolonged stress, producing extra cortisol, can also shut down insulin production.

The great problem with diabetes is not so much the control of the immediate situation – that is, the rise in blood sugar or hyperglycaemia, which causes the thirst, bladder frequency, exhaustion and fatigue, and poor response to infection. It is the long-term complications that come with it, even with reasonable control of the sugar. These are mostly the cardiovascular complications, which are due to the spiralling atherosclerosis and subsequent damage to the arteries and blood flow. There is an inevitable rise in cholesterol, especially as a result of the use of insulin, which of itself increases blood cholesterol. Coronary atherosclerosis will result, and in time: sudden death from coronary thrombosis; in the brain, strokes; in the eyes, retinal damage and later on blindness; and in the limbs, peripheral vascular disease and gangrene.

So where, you may be asking, does hypothyroidism come into all this? Well, here is a list of symptoms. Obesity, weakness and fatigue, constipation, muscle aches and pains, frequent infections, pruritus (itching), slow wound healing, high cholesterol and large babies. These are symptoms of diabetes; but you will also have noted all are common to hypothyroidism as well. The fact is, apart from the high blood sugar and sugar in the urine, there is a remarkable overlap in the symptoms of diabetes and hypothyroidism.

If that is the case, what happens if you treat diabetes with thyroid replacement? Dr Broda Barnes showed some 30 years ago that if you did this, all the symptoms improved with the only exception being the raised blood sugar. Wound healing improves, weight is lost, energy levels improve, cholesterol falls, and best of all the atherosclerosis is stopped.

One other important finding is that people who are in line for inheriting diabetes have the onset of it delayed, and benefit immeasurably by avoiding the potentially fatal cardiovascular complications.

The conclusions we can now draw are that:

1. If you have diabetes, especially the late-onset variety, you are certain to benefit from thyroid support.

2. If you have hypothyroidism and don't treat it, you are more likely to develop the NIDD kind of diabetes, sooner than you otherwise would have done.[1]

3. So, any patient with either diabetes or hypothyroidism may well find themselves troubled with both. Care must be taken to check out thyroid status if you have diabetes, and if your thyroid is down, proper investigations must be made for diabetes and special attention must be paid to diet and weight.

Chapter Fifteen

The Thyroid and Cholesterol

Since the evidence is quite overwhelming of the close link between thyroid hormones and cholesterol, and the part each plays in atherosclerosis, I really think we should examine this in more detail. These days, cholesterol is regarded as the great assassin; a multi-million dollar drug industry has been built around reducing cholesterol, together with a vast dieting industry for the same purpose; all terribly mistaken and in direct conflict with the evidence.

The story goes back to before 1900 when pathologists in Vienna noticed that hypothyroid patients were suffering more heart attacks than the general population – though these were much less common then than now. They noticed that patients who had had their thyroid removed developed atherosclerosis, with damaged, furred up arteries – especially the coronary arteries. All this was reported in 1895, would you believe. But it was ignored and forgotten by all but a few dedicated doctors, notably Eugene Hertoghe and later Broda Barnes.

In 1933, Friedland[1] published a 5 year study, where he reported that rabbits, which, being vegetarian, do not have much cholesterol at all, when actually given it developed atherosclerosis – but this was prevented if they were given thyroid hormone. It had also been found that removing the rabbits' thyroids had a similar effect; they too started to have high blood levels of cholesterol and developed atherosclerosis.[2] This work was confirmed by Broda Barnes.[3]

The great cholesterol scandal really took off with a vast study in the early 1980s, when the National Institutes of Health in the USA announced, very loudly and shrilly, that cholesterol was a major factor in heart attacks, that reducing cholesterol reduced heart attacks, and (wait for it) that there was a marvellous drug that did just this. A number of doctors challenged these findings[4, 5, 6, 7] but were ignored for their pains, even though statins were making people ill.

High cholesterol firstly is not necessarily caused by what is today seen as bad eating, and secondly is not necessarily the cause of atherosclerosis. What causes atherosclerosis is hypothyroidism allied particularly to smoking. Consider this:

1. The body makes 80% of all the cholesterol present.

2. Cholesterol may come from any source, not just polyunsaturated fats; it can be made from proteins and carbohydrates.

Even with a high cholesterol diet, a normal thyroid function will keep it within bounds. Barnes reported in 1972 that a low fat diet in the war years had not protected arteries from atherosclerosis. Other researches have confirmed these findings; indeed, much earlier in 1940, Bodansky and Bodansky in their book, *The Biochemistry of Disease*,[8] wrote that hypothyroidism can be diagnosed purely by a raised cholesterol level. As it still can.

It is amazing, disgraceful and scandalous that these findings, and there are too many to list, are ignored by doctors today. Instead of properly looking for low thyroid function, and making the correct connections, all modern doctors seem to be interested in is expensive, and often tiresome, drugs to lower cholesterol. Which, by and large they do, ignoring the actual cause.

What do we need cholesterol for? Why does the body go to the bother of making it? Well, it is needed for proper development of the brain and nervous system. It is needed in fertilisation and foetal life. In the skin, it produces vitamin D (for our bones) under the action of sunlight. It is the basic structure of the adrenal cascade of hormones, as we saw earlier.

Here is something else on which to ponder. Atherosclerosis actually begins before cholesterol gets involved; the build up of cholesterol to excessive levels is part of the process *after* the initial degeneration of the lining of the artery begins.

No one questions that high cholesterol levels increase the risk of atherosclerosis, but this is certainly not the whole story. It has been suggested recently that a significant reduction of cholesterol may well be associated with an increased risk of depression, suicide and murder. So therefore the approach should be, must be, to get the eating right. Fats are not the great evil, though you should stick to unsaturated fats where you can. Keep your weight well under control ensuring that the refined carbohydrates are properly rationed. Ensure that you have proper defences against free radicals – vitamin C is one excellent way of doing this; say 2 grams per day. Ensure there are enough of the B group vitamins and also vitamin E, another weapon against free radicals. But above all, remember that your thyroid status may be under threat – from environmental pollutants and toxins and, in this day and age, simply from heredity and the passage of time.

While we are on the subject of survival we must have a few words about homocysteine. This is an amino acid that is toxic and dangerous and is made where there is faulty metabolism of methyl compounds in our diet. It turns out that higher than normal levels have a close relation to the arterial damage of atherosclerosis, and hence heart attacks and strokes; and they are found where thyroid metabolism is running low. Much more than cholesterol, it predicts our risk of death from these diseases and the risk of its presence is increased by lack of the B group vitamins and the mineral zinc. Read Patrick Holford and Dr James Braly's book *The H Factor* for the full frightening details.

Chapter Sixteen

The Thyroid and Depression

Depression causes untold misery and destroys lives. Perhaps one in five people will suffer from it some time in their lives. A huge industry has arisen around the treatment of depressive illness and psychiatrists are gainfully employed in their thousands. Whether it is more widespread than it was is perhaps difficult to answer. There are more of us to be depressed; we have more to be depressed about; and we are more likely to seek help. But there certainly *seem* to be more people troubled by depression, and the great panoply of antidepressant medication tells its own story.

Before having a look at thyroid deficiency and its link to depression, we should learn a bit about it, and how it is caused and why. People who are depressed are sad, unmotivated most of the day and are usually worse in the morning. They sleep poorly, and wake up tired; they feel worthless; they have a poor self-image. They may eat more or less and put on or lose weight. Sir Winston Churchill used to call it his Black Dog. In his case, as with many, it was self-limiting: probably an extra cigar and brandy banished it…

Of the two main kinds of depression, we can recognise *endogenous depression* and *exogenous* or reactive depression. The first comes from within ourselves; the second comes from outside factors. The exogenous form is not so much a medical problem, since the change of circumstance for the better will relieve the depression. In fact, the difference is that the winning lottery ticket cheers up the reactive depressed patient at once; whereas the other will probably be unmoved or convinced that his new wealth will be his undoing. So we are going to deal only with the first sort, that is, endogenous depression. Some actual dysfunction in the brain is at work; and we may select five main groups of problems causing the depression. These are:

1. *Psychosocial*. This stems from possibly deep-laid psychological patterns in the personality, and may need long-term psychiatric reprogramming to correct it. An unhappy or abused childhood may well lay the foundations.

2. *Organic disease*. An illness of the brain itself affects its function. This could be something like a tumour, or a degenerative disease, or a generalised illness of the central nervous system, damaging the brain itself – Parkinson's disease, for example, or Alzheimer's.

3. *General systemic illness*. Constant pain, or loss of bodily function or unrelenting arthritis, will inevitably cause a reaction in mood to cause depression.

4. *Genetic*. There may be an inherited pattern of thinking and mood disturbance: the way one is 'wired up' as it were. Several members of the same family may all suffer in this way.

5. ***Biochemical***. The subtle mechanisms which maintain mood may not work as they should, and indeed may oscillate from one extreme to another. In the more severe forms, there are people who are really extremely cheerful, inappropriately so, for some of the time, and then relapse into the blackest gloom. We used to call these manic-depressives; the modern term is bipolar disorder.

We need now to look at these biochemical mechanisms which maintain our mood, and whose failure results in depressive illness. These are undertaken by neurotransmitter hormones, which enable brain cells to communicate with, and influence, each other. There seem to be a large number of these, but we shall look at the most important, those most likely to be influenced by failure of thyroid hormone function. Mood depends on the release of these neurotransmitters by brain cells, which are received by the receptors at the post-synaptic plate of the next nerve cell. Excess will over-stimulate mood to cause a manic state; a deficiency will work in reverse and cause depression. The whole biochemistry is very subtle and easily upset.

Recent work on the causes of depression has focused on stress hormones. The adrenocorticotrophic release hormone (CRH) is produced in response to stress, by the hypothalamus; passing down the pituitary stalk, it activates the pituitary gland to produce the adrenocorticotrophic hormone (ACTH). This stimulates adrenal cortex activity, in particular to produce cortisol. It has been found that the CRH can be made elsewhere other than in the hypothalamus – that is, in several sites within the brain. Persistent and undue secretion of CRH in unrelenting stress situations is thought to affect the seat of emotion, the hippocampus, directly, and degrade its function, inevitably promoting depression.

The recognised causes of neurotransmitter failure are these.

1. ***Increased α2-adrenergic receptors***. These receptors respond (or bind) to noradrenaline (called norepinephrine in the USA), which acts in the brain as a neurotransmitter, being secreted by certain specialist brain cells. The noradrenaline passes to the hippocampus (the part of the brain especially concerned with the maintenance of mood) and promotes mood elevation. If any mechanism inhibits the production of the noradrenaline it will result in depression. Loss of proper levels of thyroid hormone or resistance to its uptake will do this. Low thyroid hormone causes extra levels or extra activity of these adrenergic receptors, hence causing depression.

2. ***Decreased β-adrenergic receptors***. On the other hand, loss of thyroid hormone activity *lessens* β-adrenergic receptors, allowing a dominance of the α2-adrenergic receptors. The overall effect is a slowing down of intracellular metabolism. As we saw, the increased density of α2-adrenergic receptors and the decreased levels in the brain of noradrenaline are one major cause of the depression seen in hypothyroid patients (and those suffering from fibromyalgia/ME/CFS).

3. ***Low serotonin***. Serotonin is a fundamental component of the neurotransmitter hierarchy, its main role being its involvement in emotional states. Receptors bind serotonin released by neurones, and the amount of serotonin produced and bound is reduced in depression. Deficiency of thyroid hormone will reduce the amount of serotonin binding. The standard therapy is the use of selective serotonin reuptake inhibitors (SSRIs), which lessen the natural

decay of the serotonin, so allowing it to remain longer in the synaptic area (that is, the area between the neurotransmitter and the receiver cell) – which therefore increases the overall concentration. This enables the mood to return to normal. Obviously then, when thyroid hormone is deficient, as soon as replacement is provided, the situation will return to normal without an SSRI.

4. ***Monoamine oxidase activity***. The noradrenaline we were looking at earlier is removed (like serotonin) by a process of deamination (removal of NH2 radical), by an enzyme called monoamine oxidase working at other synaptic areas. This enzyme activity increases with low thyroid states, so more of the noradrenaline is degraded – which then lowers the mood. No longer much used, the monoamine oxidase inhibitors (MAOIs) group of antidepressants work to lessen the activity of the enzyme, so increasing the available noradrenaline and thus making us more cheerful. Where there is a reduced thyroid function the supplementation of thyroid hormone will have the same effect on the enzyme system without using an MAOI.

5. ***Deficient physical activity***. Low emotional states can be lifted by regular physical activity. The problem is that a poorly acting thyroid doesn't motivate one to exercise; but many patients have found this secret, and have improved their thyroid activity and their mood by regular workouts. Of course, if you have both low adrenal reserve and/or severe hypothyroidism, exercise should be worked up to slowly.

All these types of depression are likely to respond to modern antidepressants, and any admission of tiredness, sadness, lack of self-worth, is more than likely to result in a course of an antidepressant. The fact is that in very many such people, the depression is actually the reflection of a disturbance in their body hormone chemistry, and correcting this disturbance may mean that psychotropic drugs don't have to be used at all. A substantial number of people presenting at the doctors with depression, somewhere between a third and one half of the total, are depressed actually because of undetected, and unsought, imbalances in their hormones. The most common is, of course, hypothyroidism.[1]

Hypothyroidism, depending on the degree of failure, length of time present, and imbalance of other hormones, presents with a gamut of symptoms. No one patient is affected quite like any other, but as we know a number of symptoms are common to most patients. Apart from those we are so familiar with, many thyroid patients do indeed suffer from depression. This lessens their drive and motivation so much that eventually they can't be bothered to seek treatment, or if they do, follow it through. The depression is an overall bleakness and sadness which may quite often lift when the weather warms up, especially if they go on holiday, when the improvement can be quite dramatic.

Any patient suffering from depression should be routinely assessed for hypothyroidism. There should be no exceptions; half to one third will be found to be hypothyroid, and as a result of treatment, their depression will begin to lift in weeks. For a short period, it is not unreasonable, though it may not be necessary, to use an antidepressant concurrently with the thyroid medication. The problem with antidepressants is that they are sometimes difficult to stop taking. Of the SSRIs, Seroxat (paroxetine) in particular has a poor reputation in this respect; Prozac (fluoxetine) has attracted unfavourable reports and moreover contains a fluoride compound. Tricyclic antidepressants (e.g. amitriptyline, imipramine) often have unpleasant sedating side effects, and the MAOIs (e.g. Parnate (tranylcypromine), Nardil (phenelzine)) clash with a number of drugs and foodstuffs. One would be inclined to suggest St John's Wort, or the combination of the omega-3 fatty acid derivative eicosapentaenoic acid (EPA) and virgin evening primrose oil (VegEPA), as altogether simpler and safer.

The question is sometimes asked: do antidepressants act against thyroid hormones? While care has to be given to *hyperthyroid* patients receiving antidepressants – they can cause hyper-excitability – in general there is no problem with the under-active thyroid patient. As I pointed out, when depression is a particular feature, an antidepressant as well may be quite useful to get things going. However, any causing sedation have to be avoided; the hypothyroid patient is already slow enough. Also, one is anxious to avoid any risk of dependence; this is because once some improvement is apparent on a chosen antidepressant, neither doctor nor patient wants to stop using it.

I think it is important to be clear about the fact that the body has to be considered as a whole. This is called holistic medicine, and all medicine should be like this. So when we consider hypothyroidism we have to consider other factors as well, or the response to the condition will not be complete.

First, there are the other hormones. Depression of the type we are considering, with a lowered metabolism underlying it, is affected by the sex hormones, cortisol output and DHEA. Without testosterone and oestrogen being on line (and therefore if necessary being supplemented), response will necessarily be incomplete. Lack of cortisol creates mental confusion, and blanking out on minimal stress, with a claustrophobic depression. Lack of DHEA seems most associated with nervousness and irritability, anxiety and loss of sex drive. Low oestrogen of itself causes in women a flat endless depression, and lack of testosterone does much the same in men, with irritability and emotional instability. Low progesterone in women creates irrational and irritable thinking and sometimes aggression with anxiety.

Secondly, underpinning the treatment we have been discussing must be proper nutrition and vitamin and mineral supplementation. Aim for plenty of fruits and vegetables, protein in modest amounts, complex (unrefined) carbohydrates, rather than sugars, starches and breads. Supplements which must be added are these: the B group vitamins, folic acid in reasonable doses, and vitamin C, 1 or 2 grams a day. Minerals must include calcium, magnesium, copper, zinc, iron and potassium.

Not only are very many depressed people actually hypothyroid and therefore easily treated without antidepressants, but also there are other disturbances of brain function that can be and often are the result of lowered metabolic activity. Cognitive loss and memory loss are common complaints – this is the 'brain fog' familiar to so many. Concentration, attention span, the ability to think quickly and the ability to memorise things, all become degraded. Until you have had the benefit of thyroid supplementation, you may well be unaware of what you are missing. You may not have realised that you weren't enjoying life as perhaps you deserve. (Poor sleep is another problem which quietly puts itself right.)

These days we are all much exercised about Alzheimer's disease, which, for whatever reason, is *getting more common.*[2] It may present as mild but inexplicable depression. Thyroid supplementation may prevent its onset and modify its progress by ensuring the optimum nutrition of the brain cells. Brain cells need oxygen, a lot of it; liothyronine (T3) is the hormone governing the passage of oxygen across the cell membrane and the proper function of the energy-producing mitochondrion in each cell. T3 receptors are found in huge profusion everywhere in the brain.

I came to the conclusion some time ago that many apparently mentally infirm people in hospitals over long periods for chronic depression, perhaps with psychotic episodes, could well have their illness laid at the door of hypothyroidism; but no-one had thought of it in their assessment, or if they had, had relied on simple tests which missed the diagnosis. We must be forever alert for ourselves, and others close to us; hypothyroid illness is common, and *common things commonly occur*.

Chapter Seventeen

The Growth Hormone Saga

It all started in 1990, when Dr Rudman slipped a research paper into the prestigious *New England Journal of Medicine*; and medicine was never quite the same again.[1] He had invited a dozen elderly gentlemen to have an injection three times a week. Six months later, all of them had become younger by about 10 years.

A result of which Dr Frankenstein would have been truly proud.

* * *

Growth hormone (also known as somatotrophin), we briefly had a look at as one of the hormones the pituitary makes. It is one of the most abundant hormones in the body and is an extraordinarily complex molecule containing 191 amino acids, no less. From the pituitary it passes through the bloodstream to the liver, which remodels it into other hormones, the chief of which is called 'insulin-like growth factor' (previously called somatomedin C). This is shortened to IGF-1. Its job? To promote and control growth. We make a great deal of it when we are young – at peak, about 2000 mcg daily; and so we turn from children to adults. By the time we are 20, however, the amount has dropped to between 200 and 400 micrograms a day. It remains at much that level until middle age; and then declines slowly, until by 70 to 80 years of age it has nearly gone, having dropped to barely 25 mcg daily.

In the adult, human growth hormone (HGH) changes its role; it oversees and controls the output of the other glands in the endocrine orchestra and promotes good health in a variety of ways. If the output from the pituitary drops particularly low early, the hapless sufferer ages before time; if the output remains brisk, ageing is delayed, and a vigorous old age may be looked forward to.

Originally, growth hormone was extracted, at great expense and at some risk, from the human pituitary, but for many years it has been synthesised in the laboratory and is called **recombinant growth hormone**. Its primary purpose has been to normalise growth in children born with a faulty pituitary gland, which fails to produce enough HGH for the body's needs. Without it children fail to grow and die at an early age. For this purpose it is still used. However, as a result of the work of Dr Rudman, a great deal of research is now being carried on to establish its function and possible use in adults.

In the normal course of events the growth hormone lasts a relatively short time in the bloodstream and is turned into IGF-1, which lasts only minutes. During that time it really has a lot of work to do and it is now clear that it plays a vital controlling role in:

- The conversion of fat to muscle.

- Tissue growth, repair and cell replacement.

- Energy levels.

- Bone strength.

- Brain activity.

- Sexual function.

- Enzyme and hormone production.

- Prevention of cancer.

- Prevention of insulin resistance.

Since it is very clear that many of the changes due to ageing are tied up with human growth hormone (HGH) production, the question is: is this inevitable as the pituitary gland ages, and can we do anything about it? The answer seems to be that the pituitary is programmed to produce less and less HGH as time passes but can produce a great deal more if it is encouraged to do so. As to why it is programmed to slow down its production of HGH, there seems to be no clear answer, but the pineal production of melatonin is involved in the equation.

We can fight back in two ways. First, we can give HGH by injection, as was done by Dr Rudman. This of course requires medical prescription and supervision. There are disadvantages to this. One is the colossal expense. HGH by injection will cost the best part of £100 per week. Other disadvantages are the risk of liver damage and raised blood pressure. Other investigators have suggested that at higher than suitable doses there is a marginally increased risk of brain tumour, congestive cardiac failure, the carpal tunnel syndrome and the condition of bone overgrowth called acromegaly ('Jaws' in the James Bond films is an example of this). However, the essence of hormone replacement is physiological dosage. Small amounts may be given with very great overall benefit. This approach is endorsed by Thierry Hertoghe in his book *The Hormone Solution*.

But the benefits of extra HGH are very numerous, and here is a list from Dr Rudman's work.

- 8.8% increase in muscle mass after 6 months.

- 14.4% loss of fat in the same time.

- Raised energy levels and an increase in exercise tolerance.

- Repair and growth of major organs.

- Increase in heart output.

- Improvement in immune response.

- Cholesterol and lipid profiles much improved.

- Regulation of the menstrual cycle.

- Increase in bone strength.

- Improved skin elasticity and wound healing.

- Re-growth of hair.

- Loss of wrinkles.

- Improvement in vision, mood, memory and sleep.

The extraordinary beneficial effects of HGH by injection and the side effects place us in a quandary; we would certainly like all these benefits, but not with these kinds of risk. Is there any alternative? Yes there is.

First, it turns out that we can do a great deal ourselves. Plenty of exercise seems to be important, particularly (funnily enough) on an empty stomach; and a proper diet low in refined carbohydrate is pretty essential. The more obese you are, the lower is your growth hormone output. The highest production of HGH, which is very uneven anyway, occurs at night. So a good nights sleep is essential.

Secondly, we can take advantage of the fact that certain compounds have the property of stimulating natural HGH production by the pituitary. They are called **secretogogues**. These contain amino acids of which the most important are glycine, L-glutamine, L-tyrosine, L-arginine and L-lysine. Also important are GABA and pyroglutamic acid. There are products combining these amino acids and other nutrients. Nutritional supplementation should include iron, calcium, iodine, zinc, and vitamins A, B and D.

There are some 40 or so products now available, costing from about \$50/£30 per month upwards, and no doubt some are better than others; if you think they are for you, check out USA websites. The great thing is, since they contain naturally occurring products they are perfectly safe and free from the risks of the HGH injection. If not as powerful as the injectable form, they are nevertheless a perfectly reasonable option, and it is possible to lift the circulating HGH to 200 or 300 mcg or so, which, though not as high, is perfectly acceptable, since the normal range is between 90 and 360 mcg in the adult. Moreover secretogogues may be used without a time limit.

I have to say that I have not used them myself and would not recommend them unless you are perfectly sure your thyroid and adrenal systems are running normally. The thyroid connection is really two-fold. Growth hormone may actually worsen hypothyroidism so that it is crucial to get your thyroid status back on line and settled for perhaps a year before using HGH or a secretogogue. The other connection is that with your thyroid and adrenal status normal your natural output of HGH is likely to be optimal. Having said that, I can see no possible objection to secretogogues as a way of maintaining health, immune response and to slow the ageing process.

As usual some authorities are buoyantly enthusiastic about their use, and some aren't. The establishment view is that HGH should not be used except in the somatotrophin deficiency syndrome (failure of a weak pituitary to produce enough HGH), in which case, only the injectable form is of any value. My own view is that the secretogogues can help and at least are perfectly safe. Even if they do not raise your HGH levels to optimum values, they may nevertheless be part of a full programme of your healthcare and I believe they have an increasing role to play.

Chapter Eighteen

For Doctors

Thyroid deficiency disease is extremely common and is a diagnosis that should be considered for a large number of apparently unrelated illnesses apart from its classical presentation. It is not at all difficult to diagnose, and the rewards of treatment extremely gratifying.

The first problem is that we have been brainwashed into thinking that hypothyroidism is *not* common – I have seen 2% quoted – whereas it may be present, at least in a subclinical form, in perhaps 30% of the population by midlife. The second fundamental problem is that our journals and specialists tell us that the diagnosis should rely on biochemical testing. The two things to make clear about this are that (i) a full clinical appraisal is quite sufficient to make the diagnosis, with or without biochemistry, and (ii) the standard tests may be extraordinarily unreliable, and give a completely false impression.

Since the condition is so common, any patient presenting in the surgery should be the subject of a mental checklist. A multiplicity of symptoms, with tiredness, lack of drive and energy, weight gain, depression, headaches, coldness, bad skin, puffy face, should at once raise an index of suspicion. Physical examination may well reveal a slow pulse, cold extremities, a low pulse pressure, periorbital oedema, a scalloped tongue, and delayed Achilles reflex; and the basal temperature simply must be asked for. Laboratory tests may not only prove unrevealing but since they may actually falsify the situation, must be carefully interpreted. In standard practice, hypothyroidism is usually decided upon by a rise in the TSH. If it *is* raised, that is helpful, but if not, this is likely to be due to down-regulation of hypothalamic response to thyroid blood levels, or poor response of the pituitary to TRH, or poor response of thyroid follicular cells in the manufacture of thyroid hormone in response to TSH. The commonest cause of low TSH is over-stimulation of the Gq/11 proteins, which suppress both TSH production and T4 production. Blood testing may reveal low T4 and low T3, not necessarily out of range, but low. If doubt exists, the 24 hour urine test, described by Baisier and Hertoghe,[1] is probably more sensitive and more accurate.

The diagnosis must therefore be essentially clinical. Thyroid support may be exhibited if there is no risk of low adrenal reserve; but this must be considered a possibility if the patient has been ill for some time and/or is more than a little troubled by their symptoms. In considering the need for adrenal support we need to understand the concept of the **general adaption syndrome** (GAS) in our response to stress and threats to our survival. This has three stages, which are self-explanatory:

Stage I is where the hypothalamus, pituitary and adrenal glands mobilise everything we've got. Adrenaline and noradrenaline to provide energy and extra muscular power for the immediate emergency; and cortisol to mobilise blood sugar and shut down unwanted body processes and prepare our system for high stress levels.

Stage II is where, if the challenge persists, the system has to organise itself at all levels to survive. This is where prolonged, that is chronic stress, shades into exhaustion, and the adrenal glands can do no more.

Stage III. Finally, the system runs down to a situation of adaptive failure.

At some point during the investigations, the levels of DHEA should be checked. High cortisol together with high DHEA suggests that the adrenals are under a high level of stress, stage I of GAS, and able to respond. High cortisol and low DHEA shows evidence of stage II of the GAS, when the response is beginning to maladapt. Low DHEA and low cortisol will suggest adrenal exhaustion. A high DHEA with a variable or low cortisol level is strong evidence that the glucocorticoid pathway from pregnenolone to cortisol is interrupted and can only be corrected by the use of cortisone. High cortisol levels may be reduced by the use of DHEA, which will suppress the over-response of adrenal function (in a dose of 25 to 50 mg daily or 7-keto-DHEA 25 mg). Pregnenolone may be used as an alternative to DHEA, usually 30 mg daily. (If blockage to cortisol manufacture is at 17-OH-Pregnenolone level, then give biotin as it helps maintain enzymatic production such as the 21-Hydroxylase enzyme.)

In the investigation of adrenal maladaption, generally serum cortisol and the Synacthen test are widely used; but these may be just as flawed as standard thyroid function tests. The salivary adrenal stress index is very much to be preferred, being more reliable; cortisol estimation in a 24 hour urine may also be helpful. Failure to provide adrenal support for the first few weeks will result in a limited response, no response at all, or actually unwanted toxic symptoms.

This may most effectively be carried out by the use of non-prescription bovine adrenal glandular concentrate; as well as providing all the adrenal hormones, it also contains the enzymes to make them. Nutri Ltd make two useful and widely available products, one without supplementary vitamins and minerals, Nutri Adrenal containing 80 grams of glandular concentrate, and one with, Nutri Adrenal Extra containing 221 grams. The dose of the former is up to 4 times daily and of the latter twice daily, both to be taken in the morning with food. (It occasionally happens that the vitamins and minerals may prove rather too much for some sensitive patients and therefore the lower dose product without supplements may be preferable.) Recourse may be made if it becomes necessary to the physiological use of hydrocortisone and prednisolone; for example, from 2.5 up to 20 mg of hydrocortisone or 2.5 to 5 mg of prednisolone, and should be provided as a sensible precaution, discontinued when the patient has shown established signs of response to thyroid hormone.

The use of low dosage cortisone replacement may be a mental hurdle both the doctor and the patient may need to surmount. It should be pointed out that the adrenals produce cortisone all the time in the resting state and significantly increased amounts in long-term stress. For acute stress, adrenaline and noradrenaline are produced but this is not relevant in this context. This cortisol production is a normal physiological response to stress and in this situation the stress is the result of being ill with hypothyroidism. Providing adrenal support in the form of glandular concentrate, cortisone or prednisolone, *in physiological doses*, is therefore not only perfectly safe but may well be mandatory. It will *not* cause adrenal suppression in these doses and may be discontinued when deemed clinically appropriate. This will occur when the adrenal function, closely tied up with, and dependent on, tissue response to thyroid hormone, is coming back to normal. Patients need to understand the rationale of treatment and careful explanation may well be necessary, although many patients these days are quite well informed.

Having established the need, if it seems appropriate, for adrenal support, the patient should be considered for other deficiencies, both hormonal and nutritional. Levels of oestrogen and progesterone in women in early middle life and beyond may be relevant and consideration should be given to the careful use of HRT. It is a matter of common experience that progesterone starts to fall off as the menopause approaches (even in the thirties), to cause worsening PMT, and heavy and/or irregular periods. Natural progesterone as a transdermal cream is most commonly more satisfactory than progestogens. Oestrogen may not be required at this stage, and an oestrogen dominance situation can be worsened by well meaning but inappropriate use of oestrogen derivatives. Approaching or passing middle life, gentlemen too must have their testosterone checked and supplemented if low, using a transdermal testosterone cream, or Restandol or Sustanon.

Many patients are slipping into multiple nutritional deficiencies, perhaps from inanition, but usually from poor absorption; a full biochemical work-up to include urea and electrolytes, together with calcium and potassium would seem essential. Multiple mineral and vitamin supplements are a must, and iron, vitamin C, B Complex, and selenium, are certainly relevant. Certain products are available which contain these raw materials all in one preparation.

The stage is now set for the use of thyroid supplementation. You have certain choices, which must be exercised. First, for patients whose blood tests may be equivocal but with a nevertheless convincing clinical diagnosis, it is effective, safe and proper to consider the use of natural glandular extracts. These are licensed as food products, and are provided by, for example, Nutri Meds (bovine or porcine sourced) or Nutri Ltd (bovine sourced) in 130 mg amounts of thyroid glandular extract. The thyroid support which will begin two or three weeks after the adrenal supplement, should be started at 1 daily in the morning with food, increasing as required to perhaps 4 daily.

The next option is the use of synthetic T4 and/or T3, or the natural desiccated thyroid. Establishment medicine has long considered that T4 is all that is necessary, and in simple early hypothyroidism, this may be true. But hypothyroidism interferes with the system's uptake of T4 and its conversion to T3, and it may be a cause of receptor resistance. The added complication of Gq/11 proteins shutting down T4 uptake and TSH production causes further difficulty. What tends to happen in patients of long-standing or previously undiagnosed thyroid dysfunction, is that the dose of T4 never seems to be right. Just as the increase of dose brings some improvement, overdose symptoms are complained of; and thyroxine estimation in the blood may show an excess. Reducing the dose relieves the overdose symptoms, but the original symptoms come creeping back. The elderly should be started on 25 mcg of T4, increasing perhaps in 28 days to 50 mcg. A ceiling may be reached at or before 100 mcg. The younger age group and those with higher body mass will usually be started on 50 mcg, with graded increase beyond 100 mcg if required. A failure to balance a patient and bring relief of symptoms (assuming the adrenal problem has been dealt with) may mean poor T4 $\rightarrow$ T3 conversion, and/or receptor resistance. At this point, T3, 10 mcg, may be introduced in partial substitution for some of the T4. It makes sound sense, and can only be good clinical practice, to use the 10 mcg of T3 (½ tablet) in the morning, or certainly no later than midday in conjunction with the T4. An amount of perhaps 20 mcg of T3 and 75 or 100 micrograms of T4 is a dose commonly decided upon. The dose of adrenal support, T3 and T4, should be monitored, initially fortnightly, with the patient providing a diary of basal temperatures, their basal pulse rate and symptomology.

I have very full experience in the use of the natural desiccated thyroid, which was used in the UK up until about 1985. A number of companies in the USA manufacture natural thyroid from bovine and porcine sources; the best known is Armour thyroid (Forest Pharmaceuticals), available in the UK on-line or through specialised pharmacies (see Appendix D). Following increasing disenchantment with thyroxine, natural thyroid is becoming more popular with patients and some doctors alike. The disenchantment with thyroxine springs from its varying potency from manufacturer to manufacturer, and similar problems occur with the American synthetic product. Although natural thyroid is widely held to be of variable potency by its critics, this is simply not true and no trials have ever supported this view. It is also very effective compared with synthetic T4. (It may be pointed out that the system's daily requirements vary dynamically and a precise dose is not actually necessary.) The natural product is a combination of T4, T3, T2 and T1, and very close indeed, and in the same proportion, to human thyroid; with very few exceptions, it is much preferred by patients. The dose is measured in grains: 1 grain is a 60 mg tablet which contains 38 mcg T4 and 9 mcg of T3. The dose is normally started with ½ a grain, building slowly by ½ a grain every 14 to 28 days to 1 or 2 grains as seems appropriate; and adjustments are made up or down subsequently. The patients are encouraged to keep a diary monitoring their pulse and basal temperatures and response to treatment more or less daily. It may be far more satisfactory to let patients decide their own dose, which, if they are fully informed, they can safely do in conjunction with you.

Two possible causes of an unsatisfactory response are, first, that a sufficiency of time must be allowed to elapse so that the system may respond to any given dose, and this may take several weeks, although a week or so should be sufficient to establish how things are going. Secondly, the level of adrenal support may need to be re-considered.

Recognition and treatment of hypothyroidism seems quite essential in view of its common occurrence as a cause of chronic illness. Undue reliance on blood tests over and above a clinical appraisal, is much to be deplored, and at the very least a trial of treatment by thyroid supplementation should be considered. The reward to the patient is a return to health; and to the doctor, not just a grateful patient, but being able to avoid expensive tests and treatments.

Chapter Nineteen

Helping Yourself

Now I want to say something again which I touched on in the Introduction. It is this. The problems created by thyroid and adrenal insufficiency are actually *very common*. So much so that it is an odds on bet that you, the reader and my patient audience, are in trouble yourself. A state of chronically lowered metabolism that this insufficiency causes is the lot of ever so many people, far, far more than doctors and endocrine specialists give credit for. So for a common illness, commonly occurring, and – let me emphasise this – easily treated, there may be no medical help available for all these uncounted numbers of people. The doctors say you are depressed, or menopausal, or old, or whatever, and you have to get on with it.

Well, as we have seen, you don't.

You *can* get the help you need. First, there are a large number of alternative health practitioners, nutritionists, kinesiologists and many others who are going to listen to you. Ever so many have listened to me, and have heard me speak, and, yes, read this book too. They know what you are going through and they will listen.

And, second, you can help yourself; take responsibility for your own health if no one else will, and *do* something. You know how to diagnose the condition now; and you know too how to treat it. Yes, but…, but, suppose I get it wrong? Okay, fair question. But we are going to use nutritional strategies: vitamins and minerals, glandular extracts. If they are not quite right, adjust the dose, taking note of the manufacturer's advice. In a month or two you will either feel better, or you won't. If you don't get any better, they will have done no harm. You will know. The anxieties about over-stimulation of the system, and the heart and so on, have little place with natural treatment, sensibly and knowledgeably used. Usually the worst that can happen is that the vitamins and minerals perhaps upset the digestion. I am not saying that some people won't shake their heads and purse their lips. But it is your life, and not theirs. Don't go on month after month, year after year, slowly getting worse. Do something. It is for you that I wrote this book, to give you the knowledge and understanding that you need.

The first part of your programme is to make the **diagnosis**. You may, after repeated visits to the doctor and repeated tests where you are told that there is nothing wrong and treatment for hypothyroidism is refused, decide to take matters into your own hands. You may wish to undertake treatment yourself on a natural basis or you may perhaps consult an alternative practitioner who will help both in the diagnosis and in the monitoring of your treatment. As I said, you will find that most alternative practitioners are very much more open to listening to you, the patient and your symptoms and will have a knowledge of natural treatments which the average establishment doctor will not have.

Many people also turn to reflexology as a means of self-help and a skilled practitioner may bring much benefit and relief to failing thyroid and adrenal function. The principle is as simple as it is unexpected; the soles of your feet (and to a lesser extent, the palms of your hands) map all the parts of the body, and any loss of function is reflected in specific areas in the feet. The use of careful massage and pressure in these areas can stimulate a target organ or gland. This is particularly relevant of course, to the endocrine system, and hence reflexology can be of great help. It may also be used diagnostically, since these areas are tender, if not painful, to applied pressure; and a reflexologist can pick up thyroid and/or adrenal problems at first examination. They can then go on to provide relief. Several successive treatments are given over a period of one or two weeks and then once or twice weekly for as long as appropriate. Patients almost always benefit from reflexology, which, seeking to stimulate the target organ to give of its best, helps to balance the system. If the degree of thyroid failure is severe or of longstanding, supplementation may be unavoidable, and the best results may be achieved through a combination of reflexology, supplementation and proper nutrition. Some of you reading this may know of my interest in reflexology, and my association with the Advanced Reflexology Training Institute. I warmly recommend that you access their website for further information (see Appendix D).

As you have read, there are steps that you must take yourself through. You may have a pretty good idea what is wrong, but it is useful and very much the right thing to do, to make a list of your symptoms and compare them with those you have read about. (You will find a full list of the symptoms in Appendix B.) When do you think it started? Was there an illness or life event which triggered things off? Review your family history and see if there is a link.

Now you must find whatever evidence there is of hypothyroidism. What are your hair and skin like? Is your face puffy? Is your skin colour perhaps a little on the yellow side? Be a bit scientific about it and check your basal temperature with care. It is well worth doing it for two or three weeks and averaging it all out. Make sure the thermometer works properly; check it against another thermometer or someone else's temperature. Three minutes in the mouth immediately on waking, before you get out of bed – having shaken it down *the night before*, and made sure it really has gone down to zero. You don't necessarily have to read it straight away – one may be a bit bleary first thing – but when you do, write it all down there and then. Make sure that you don't have a cold or flu coming on, or that you don't have a sore throat or sinus infection, or dental abscess – all these things will raise your temperature and make the basal reading invalid. You will remember that if you are of the fair sex, you have a five or six day window from the beginning of your period each month in which to take your temperature, starting on day 2. Your normal basal temperature should be above 97.6°F / 36.8°C. The correct figures are 98.4°F or 37°C. Normal, or slightly above normal temperatures will be present in hyperthyroidism. Below the lower limit of the range, it is more than likely that you have a lowered metabolism due to hypothyroidism. The only other causes of temperatures below these limits are malnutrition, liver failure, hypothermia and alcoholism. If you have had 'a good drink' the night before, discount your temperature in the morning. It's useful at the same time to take your pulse as a base line since, on successful treatment, a rise of pulse may be the first signal of success.

As far as the pulse goes, if you find difficulty in taking it (in the indentation in your wrist below the thumb) you can get a pulseometer from the chemist, which will count it for you. If you are going to do it yourself, count the number of beats in a minute or if you are late for the train, the number of beats in ½ minute and double it. Write it down. Your normal resting pulse is likely to be somewhere between 65 and 75 beats per minute. During the day it may well rise into the 80s or beyond, especially if it has been 'one of those days'. A morning pulse rate of 65 or less is certainly slow and may be further evidence. On the other hand, a pulse over 90 suggests over-activity.

From your own history of your illness, your family history and your basal temperature, you should be able to make a valid diagnosis yourself; or present enough evidence to convince your doctor. Your problems, of course, may not end there. His reaction may vary from sympathetic understanding to outright rejection.

You should be able to persuade him of the need for a blood test. Most commonly you will be offered the TSH test. Although widely regarded among doctors as excellent and reliable, it has two flaws which may torpedo the whole thing. You will remember that a raised TSH indicates a poorly responding – and therefore poorly functioning – thyroid. Problem is that TSH production may be lowered by a pituitary gland (or hypothalamus) affected by a low thyroid state and therefore not responding as it should to low thyroid hormone levels in the blood. TSH production is also lowered by the Gq/11 proteins over-responding, owing to environmental toxins such as fluoride and aluminium, as we saw earlier. So the TSH may come back in the normal range, or even low.

The other flaw lies in interpretation. Laboratories have wide variations in their normal ranges (even in the NHS) and the tests sometimes are really not very sensitive. Worse, doctors may have their own interpretation, which may not be right. I have seen figures of 5 or 6 units regarded as normal, but most workers in the field have come to believe that a lower figure should arouse a high index of suspicion; indeed anything over 2.5 units. The USA has recently reduced the upper limit of their reference range to 3.1, which is certainly an improvement; this has so far been inexplicably ignored in the UK. You may at this point want to have a look at the chart showing interpretation of TSH blood test results at the end of this chapter. If you do have a test done, ask for the figures so that you can take them home and relate them to the chart.

The scenarios you have to consider are these:

1. I'm not even going to bother going to the doctor; I think I can sort this myself.

2. The doctor says no to the blood test, and come back in six months.

3. The doctor does a blood test, which comes back 'normal'; he says, 'Come and see me again in six months.'

4. The blood test comes back abnormal showing an absent or very low TSH if you're over-active, and an above range TSH if you are hypothyroid. This should be diagnostic. But your doctor may suggest scenario 5, or go right away for 6.

5. Further tests are done, which will lead to 6.

6. Treatment will be started at once: thyroxine for hypothyroidism or neomercazole for hyperthyroidism

Before thinking about thyroid and adrenal supplementation, we must prepare the ground. This means getting your nutrition right and doing everything you can to promote for yourself a **healthy lifestyle**. Remember what I said about the environment, and consider the positive side of the coin. Ensure that your eating is healthy. You really do have to cut out the junk foods with their frightful list of additives, the E numbers, the monosodium glutamates. Reduce and eventually stop smoking and consider your alcohol intake. Wherever you can, go for the organic foods. Ensure there is a proper balance between your carbohydrates, proteins and fats; reduce your refined carbohydrates – sugars and starches – as far as possible in favour of complex carbohydrates, i.e. fruits and vegetables (the next chapter is about this). You should not avoid fats; contrary to popular belief, fats do not necessarily make you fat, and, unsaturated fats in particular are vital for so many of our body's complex systems. Just go for moderation.

Every effort has to be made to *reduce day to day stress* in your life – easily said, I admit. Let laughter into your life. Before I go onto vitamin and mineral supplementation, a word about sleep, dieting and exercise.

Sleep

For both thyroid and adrenal health, and for good health generally, you must do whatever you can to ensure a good night's sleep. It may be easier said than done, but if changing your eating habits, pillow, mattress, room, *partner*, does not work, then there are many natural remedies available, not excluding enough exercise to make you tired.

Dieting

Calorie restriction can easily reduce your metabolic rate 20% in a fortnight, so that while you can lose weight restricting calories below your requirements, your metabolism – your thyroid – slows down to compensate. What you need to do is a) restore thyroid levels to normal and b) exercise.

Exercise

Exercise is absolutely vital for all sorts of reasons, and I cannot emphasise its importance enough. Yoga and gentle stretching first thing in the morning are an excellent way to get the blood flowing to all the glands and to get things going. Take good regular aerobic exercise and I am quite happy if you get it with regular walking. You may have to progressively work up to this to avoid over-stressing your damaged metabolism, especially if the adrenal problem is quite marked.

Vitamin and Mineral Supplements

For reasons I have some hesitation in putting forward, but which may have a close relation to the pharmaceutical industry worldwide, there has been formed in recent years a body called Codex Alimentarius, which has allied itself to the World Health Organisation (WHO) and the World Food Organisation (WFO) to discourage the sale of nutritional supplements on a broad front. Some idea of what is going on may be gained by reading their aims. 'Statements on the curative effects of vitamins and other natural remedies will be barred and made a *punishable offence*' (my italics), and further; 'in future the distinction between a foodstuff and a medicine will be made by' – *wait for it* – 'the pharmaceutical industry itself and not by governments.' This outrageous affront to clinical and individual freedom is another example of the dead hand of the medical establishment, allied to the giants of the pharmaceutical industry. Following a great deal of protest, legal moves have led to a lessening of the impact of the new regulations, but the threat remains. I believe we should continue to resist these disgraceful rules. (See website in Appendix D.)

I must tell you now that optimum levels of mineral and vitamin intake are essential. Optimum levels are not the same as the RDA (recommended daily allowance), which are *minimum* amounts. First to concern us is the B complex of vitamins. Your energy metabolism is critically dependent on vitamin B_1 (thiamine); your nervous system (especially as regards depression) on vitamin B_6 (pyridoxine). Equally important is folic acid, a deficiency of which may actually lower body temperature and even cause some hypothyroid symptoms. Vitamin B deficiency will cause an intolerance to thyroid hormone so that it is clear that it's important to supplement B vitamins when giving thyroid supplements. Vitamin E intake should be somewhere between 400 and 800 iu (international units) and the addition of calcium 1000 to 1500 mg and magnesium 300 mg daily is desirable. Other trace minerals include boron, selenium, manganese and iron, which you will easily obtain in a multi-mineral preparation from your chemist. I have covered this in detail in the chapter on treatment.

Environment

We now have to worry about the negative side of the environment. Some of this you are already prepared for, but I will make this as complete as possible.

Iodine is essential for the manufacture of thyroid hormone, and can easily become deficient with imbalanced diets. You need 150 to 300 mcg daily, but not more. I have referred to this in Chapter Seven.

Lithium blocks thyroid hormone release, and its manufacture. Lithium finds wide use in the treatment of anxiety and depression, and you must ask your specialist to help you tail it off where thyroid deficiency is suspected.

Bromine is one of the four halogens (iodine, bromine, chlorine and fluorine in ascending order); these can compete with the iodine at receptor sites. It has long been used in the make-up of sedatives; any sedative containing bromine must be stopped.

Growth hormone (GH) is properly used to promote correct growth in children with pituitary deficiency. In adults, however, it has been used as an overall anti-ageing hormone. This, at great expense, works to some degree but it may have some unwelcome side effects as we saw earlier, and has been shown to worsen untreated hypothyroidism.

Fluoride compounds block iodine uptake and are enzyme poisons. I have dealt with this at some length earlier. Let me just say, drink where you can fluoride-free water, avoid fluoride-containing toothpastes, and remember that tea grows in fluoride rich soils and is an unexpected source of daily fluoride.

Anti-depressants: One particular offender is fluoxetine, which contains fluoride and thus also impairs thyroid metabolism. So do the tricyclic and monoamine oxidase inhibitors, which have suppressant effects on thyroid hormone uptake.

Dioxins and PCBs I also mentioned earlier since they interfere with thyroid hormone manufacture.

Other substances: Here is a list of some others substances which also interfere with thyroid hormone manufacture:

> Resorcinol (from millet)
> Thiocyanates (from barbiturates)
> Sulphonamides (from antibiotics)
> Amiodarone (which regulates heart action)
> Brassica family (cabbage and sprouts) contain thiouracil
> Coffee
> Alcohol

* * *

Where you are faced with scenarios 1, 2 & 3 (on page 207), you must decide whether to treat yourself or seek alternative treatment. If thyroxine is started, monitor your progress and the basal temperature, pulse and your symptoms. Failure to respond means: (i) the dosage is not right; (ii) you are unresponsive to synthetic thyroxine; (iii) you have low adrenal reserve.

You must be sure to keep your diary regularly and be prepared to adjust the dose yourself, based on this and how you feel, without waiting for blood tests which may well say one thing, while you may feel quite another. In short, have the confidence that *you* know best.

On these treatment regimes you will improve and during the coming weeks, the symptoms that have pulled you down for so long, will begin to recede. Your energy levels will improve, the terrible tiredness will be replaced with a new urge to get up and do things – but don't rush it, give it time – and you will feel warmer (but don't expect your basal temperature to become normal; it takes quite a while to rise and usually levels off a little below normal). The first sign that you are beginning to respond to the treatment will be a rise in your morning (basal) pulse rate, which will rise to the upper 60s or lower 70s beats per minute.

Your basal temperature will also rise but take its time about doing so, and as I said earlier, it is unlikely to become textbook normal. A brisk rise of temperature, approaching normal, may actually mean the thyroid supplementation is becoming too much and considered with your other symptoms, may indicate that a reduction of dosage should be made. This can also be the result of a toxic effect developing from excess thyroid hormone not being properly metabolised, so, in addition to reducing the dose, it might be right to increase your adrenal support. Furthermore, do remember that your temperature and pulse can go up and down on a daily basis, for all sorts of reasons, particularly of course, if you have a cold. Also, remember the basal temperature for women who are menstruating undergoes a cyclical change during the month. You will (joyously) find weight beginning to go; you will lose the muzzy thinking, the depressed mood, the headaches. Not only will you have done so much to restore your health; you will also have taken decisive steps in the prevention of atherosclerosis, of raised blood pressure and sudden death due to heart disease or stroke. You will have extended your life and given yourself a new vigour to enjoy it.

You haven't quite finished yet though. Just as your thyroid began to let you down, so may your other hormones. The ones that we really need to worry about are, for the ladies, oestrogen and progesterone, and all I want to say now is, think about getting your levels checked. If you have any menopausal symptoms be prepared for replacement therapy for one or both, using where possible natural products in favour of the synthetic. For the lads, testosterone can start to fail at almost any time after mid-life, and this should be checked and corrected. Likewise DHEA levels should be checked, and, as you have read, they are simple to correct.

Many hormone deficiencies correct themselves to a degree when your thyroid status becomes normal, but in the early stages of treatment other supplements may certainly have their place, and may have to be continued.

I suppose the biggest barrier to self-help is a crisis of confidence. Dare you treat yourself? Often, being ill for years undermines your self-confidence anyway, making it more difficult to decide which way to go. It is very helpful to have a practitioner with whom to share your decisions, but learn as much as possible about the problem yourself; with knowledge comes your conviction. The food supplement products I have been talking about are really perfectly safe used thoughtfully and sensibly – as much as any nutritional supplements available from chemists and health shops. You really owe it to yourself to cast off the shackles of an illness that has left you, perhaps for years, in a prison.

Many doctors simplistically think that thyroid disease can be diagnosed, and even worse, its treatment can be governed, by testing only TSH levels. For many reasons, and many are shown in this book, the blood tests may not show the true picture and it is quite wrong to rely on them alone. The standard interpretation of blood tests means that a very large number of patients remain undiagnosed. The format below is more applicable than the standard textbook interpretation and it may help you to understand your test results. [1, 2, 3, 4]

Figure 16. The interpretation of TSH blood test results

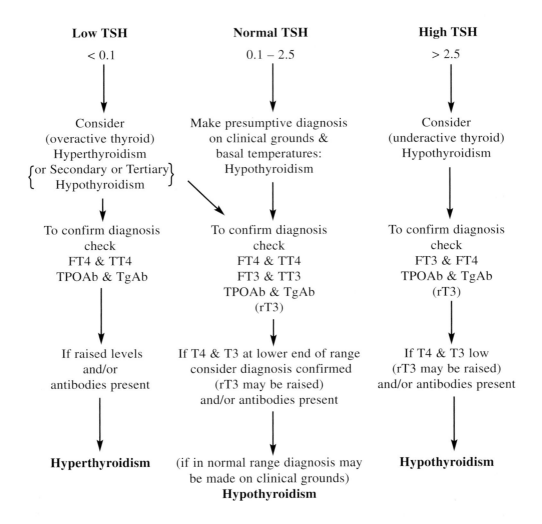

Abbreviations
< less than   > more than
FT4 – Free thyroxine   FT3 – Free liothyronine   TSH – Thyroid stimulating hormone
TT4 – Total thyroxine   TT3 – Total liothyronine   rT3 – Reverse T3
TPOAb – Thyroperoxidase antibodies   TgAb – Antithyroglobulin antibodies

14 Day Report

Week Ending:

DAY	MEDICATION	DOSAGE	TEMP AM	TEMP PM	PULSE AM	PULSE PM	OBSERVATIONS	1-10 RATING	ACTIVITIES
1									
2									
3									
4									
5									
6									
7									

14 Day Report

Week Ending:

DAY	MEDICATION	DOSAGE	TEMP AM	TEMP PM	PULSE AM	PULSE PM	OBSERVATIONS	1-10 RATING	ACTIVITIES
8									
9									
10									
11									
12									
13									
14									

Chapter Twenty

Losing Weight

– Refined Carbohydrate, The Great Enemy

There is a problem in the Western world: people are getting more overweight year by year and the death rate from obesity-related illnesses rises inexorably. And this is in spite of greater awareness of these health risks, and different diets by the dozen. Yet still the problem gets worse.

What is wrong? Why are there so many diets – and still our weight remains out of control?

As we have seen, and are very much aware ourselves, weight gain is a feature of hypothyroid illness that causes endless physical and emotional stress and applies to many more people than the medical profession realises. Without ensuring proper thyroid function, we stand no chance of losing weight, unless somebody shuts us up in a box for a couple of months. But with metabolism coming back on line, the wonderful news is that now weight *can* be lost, without pain and torment, and actually stay off. What I am going to say now applies to dieting both in low metabolic states and to people who are simply overweight.

There has grown up a fundamental misunderstanding about eating, worsened by what seems to be deliberate misinformation by healthcare practitioners and food manufacturers.

Even when you are perfectly healthy – though overweight – and thyroid function, and hence metabolism, are normal, dieting will inevitably produce a (hopefully) temporary fall in your metabolic processes which may soon drop to something like 75% of normal. Your system, recognising that the overall energy intake is dropping, compensates by lowering your thyroid output, so that you burn fewer calories than before. Everybody knows that in the first few days of brisk dieting, you may actually lose pounds; but then it all seems to slow down and plateau off. It is the thyroid that does this. The mechanism is multifactorial: one way it works is that the TSH level drops, the hypothalamus recognising that the energy stores need to be conserved in what it sees as a famine situation, and instructs the pituitary-thyroid axis accordingly. As we saw earlier, another mechanism is the production of reverse T3 (thus reducing normal T3), which of course has the same metabolism lowering effect.

Anyhow, it all slows down. One way you can fight this is to exercise, adding insult to injury by leaping about with less disposable energy to draw upon. This of course is the point; the energy deficit is found from metabolising calories from the fat stores. If the dieting is too extreme, the system will start to break down (catabolise) protein from muscle tissue, which is a bad thing. The slowing down of thyroid output can be compensated for by increasing the thyroid supplement dosage. I noted earlier on that it seems that T2 has a significant effect on the metabolism of fat without involving the protein in muscle, and new products are available to exploit this. I have no knowledge of their use, however; I mention it only for the sake of completeness.

When weight has been lost, the end of the dieting programme should be a progressive, not abrupt, return to normal, to allow your metabolism to speed back up to normal gradually, keeping a hands on approach to your thyroid problems as you do so.

Let us start by examining why we get fat. People become overweight by eating too much. Well, this has to be true of course; but the reverse doesn't follow; some people who *don't* overeat also get fat.

There can be no doubt that in 'developed' countries we all eat more than we were intended to and different foods from those for which evolution designed us. But many people eat perfectly reasonably and still get fat; equally, many overeat and remain normal in weight. Deliberate overeating – being simply greedy – will overload the mechanisms which regulate our weight. The problems here are psychological and may be deep-rooted in our upbringing; or we may over-indulge to provide comfort in the pleasurable activity of eating. Dieting, or any sort of imposed control, may well be impossible. There are not that many people like this, but if they want help their attitudes can be changed, even by simple medication to control appetite. The condition of morbid obesity can result from a failure of the stomach to release the hormones gastrin and leptin, which tell us when we are full, or a failure of the brain to respond to them. When this happens, you will continue to feel hungry however much you have eaten.

Probably though, the underlying problem of a great many people, often those with really severe weight problems, lies in their inability to process their chief foodstuff properly. And this is the unrecognised enemy, the evil around us every day of our lives. *NOT* fat. Not protein. But *REFINED CARBOHYDRATE*. It is refined carbohydrate that makes us fat, and refined carbohydrate that imperils our success in losing weight. Farmers have known for 5,000 years that to fatten their hogs, you give them carbohydrate – mostly as corn. Not fat.

Refined carbohydrates are a high energy source. Because they are low in fibre, they are easily and rapidly digested. Within a very short time, they are converted to glucose within the bloodstream and high levels are reached very rapidly. Since there is little chance that this energy will be used quickly, insulin is secreted by the pancreas to lower the blood sugar, and the glucose is converted to glycogen to be stored by the liver. The glycogen is re-converted back to glucose on demand, over a 24 hour span, so that it acts as a short-term energy source. If glycogen stores are full, the glucose is converted instead to fat and transported to the tissues for long-term storage. This long-term energy storage may become excessive, but with continuous high energy foodstuffs there is nowhere else for the energy – this means calories – to go. So we get fatter and fatter.

The problem is the excess energy input, with no mechanism to slow its absorption. The slowing of absorption is carried out by fibre; the more fibre there is, the less the surge of glucose into the bloodstream. Refined carbohydrates are low in fibre; sugar, for example has none at all. Fats and proteins are less rapidly digested and the biochemical mechanisms for their disposal are more complex; also, our capacity for a high fat or high protein intake is limited. We get full quickly on fatty things; we cannot eat more than modest amounts. Carbohydrates are different; we can eat a great excess of many common refined carbohydrates, and still ask for more. Chocolate for example!

There exists now a terrible confusion about fats. Over the last 30 years or so, we have been taught that consuming fat produces fat in our bodies and so the less we eat the better. As with everything in life, it is only moderation that is required for good health. When it was discovered that high blood levels of triglycerides and cholesterol, the end product of eating fat, were associated with an increase in atherosclerotic disease – coronary thrombosis, high blood pressure, strokes – we were brainwashed by healthcare practitioners and food manufacturers into eating less fat. The correctness of this association is really not clear at all. For example, people get these illnesses with normal cholesterol and triglycerides, and the Americans, who now mostly eat low-fat foods, have a higher mortality from heart disease than ever before. I pointed out already that 80% of the cholesterol in the body is actually manufactured by the body itself. What has been learnt in recent years is that essential fatty acids are required to maintain our body's well-being and without them we will be more inclined to suffer from heart disease. I'm not saying that we should throw caution to the winds; simply that things must be kept in perspective. As you will have learnt earlier in this book, low thyroid function will produce high cholesterol and increase the risk of coronary atherosclerosis regardless of your low fat diet.

All this has become increasingly blurred in the public mind – and in the minds of healthcare practitioners – with the weight problem, so that now we all believe that if we eat less fat, we'll get thin. But it doesn't work as it is supposed to. Most of us are just as overweight as before. That is not to say that a low-calorie, low-fat diet will not cause weight loss; it is perfectly clear that any diet made up in any way which contains fewer calories per day than our body uses, will result in weight loss. Of course it will. But this is an artificial construct; it may be difficult to do, and impossible to continue without some degree of malnutrition and of course down-regulation of the metabolism.

Proteins fall into a different category. Proteins are the building blocks of our tissues. The constant repair and renewal of our tissues requires proteins – meat, fish, eggs, pulses – and protein is essential to our eating. Protein, however, may be turned into glucose by a complex process and supply energy for living. That's why somebody on a hunger strike gets thinner and thinner; their body protein is being stripped and converted to glucose. Reducing your protein intake is another way of lessening your overall energy intake and, of course, as part of a low-calorie diet, will work. But as we know, it is obviously all wrong to do this since the weight lost will then include loss of muscle mass.

So we come back to the arch-villain of the whole story. Refined carbohydrates, (note *'refined'*) of which the worst is sugar. People don't realise that it is actually addictive; you become tolerant, dependent, and even feel ill without it. Patrick Holford is at pains to point this out and has suggested an excellent approach in his book *The Holford Low GL Diet*. Complex carbohydrates are a different story. These are fruits and vegetables. They contain more or less fibre; the more fibre, the slower the digestion and absorption and, therefore, the lower the amount of glucose surge and the lower the risk of it turning into fat. Refined carbohydrate produces energy, but we usually eat more than we can cope with, and fat is the result. The fact is that if we all ate less refined carbohydrate, more proteins, and a *modest* amount of fat, we should lose weight – whether we are actively dieting or not. OK, with some weight problems it is certainly going to take longer than if some sort of calorie control is used as well, but you can lose weight without calorie restriction by restricting only the carbohydrates. And that can ensure that the weight stays off without effort.

It seems that some people can deal with carbohydrates better than others. This concept of carbohydrate sensitivity may be new to you and, sadly, to many doctors. Most people without significant weight problems have an average carbohydrate sensitivity; that is, they can process them without the glucose excess turning into body fat unduly easily; probably, they eat normal amounts. Some people can eat as much as they like and, seemingly, get away with it. Tends to apply to the young, rather.

I'm concerned with the people with carbohydrate sensitivity. You may be one of them. You may not be able to deal with more than a small, or modest, amount of glucose surge – from refined carbohydrate – without it turning into fat. I have seen over the years many people with terrible obesity. While a combination of factors may apply, these folk are suffering from excessive sensitivity to refined carbohydrates. (Because of the strain to the pancreas, many are, or will become, diabetic.) The solution to the problem may be not dieting in the traditional sense at all, with calorie restriction watchfully applied, but with carbohydrate restriction. We must adopt a holistic approach, using several different methods. All at once, if necessary; so there will probably be partial calorie restriction applied a few days a week, together with a more or less strictly applied control to the refined carbohydrate intake all the time. I think it is important to take a break from carbohydrate dieting pretty often, say at the weekends, with no restrictions except commonsense.

So, what are these refined carbohydrates, and how much restriction do we mean?

Refined carbohydrates are the high glycaemic foodstuffs. We are talking about sugar, bread, cakes, biscuits, pasta (sorry), white rice, most fruit juices and fizzy drinks (not low calorie ones, but then you really want to avoid chemical laden drinks anyway), cereals and jams. Bread must be carefully watched; the action of ptyalin in your saliva converts the starch into sugar before you even swallow it. Stoneground flour is preferable to other kinds. The carbohydrate intake should be between 40 and 60 grams a day. This isn't a lot. Many foods when subjected to an industrialised process to become 'convenience foods', have carbohydrate added. A glance at the shelves in the supermarket reveals that, however *low-fat* things are, nearly everything contains sugar; even a can of beans.

All the meats and fish are excellent. Vegetables are all satisfactory, but potatoes have much starch, which is rapidly turned to sugar in the blood, and peas and parsnips may surprise you too. Fruit is high, but especially when raw, contains fibre which slows absorption.

There are many books available about foods and their glycaemic index containing some wonderful recipes too. It is worth buying one to help you plan your daily food intake.

Last word. It is best not to consider any form of weight loss programme until your metabolism has come back on line, as you will be unable to lose weight consistently and maintain the loss. Although you could just cut back on one or two of the extra refined carbohydrates you have daily...

Some points to consider on a weight loss regime

1. When you are on your days off calorie restriction, don't think about calories or count them.

2. Eat less than 60 grams of carbohydrate daily, but not less than 40 grams. Too little carbohydrate can give you a headache.

3. Eat what you want, when you are hungry – up to your carbohydrate allowance. But, don't eat unless you need to.

4. Multi-mineral supplements are highly desirable and you must pay special regard to vitamins of the B complex and take 1 to 2 grams of vitamin C per day.

5. Don't worry if you plateau sometimes. Use a tape measure as well as scales. Fat is still burning off, but protein rebuilds muscle that may have been lost by previous poor eating, lack of exercise, and episodes of severe calorie restriction in crash dieting – and,

volume for volume, muscle weighs seven times as much as fat. The way your clothes fit is more important than what the scales say.

6. When you are at the weight you want, increase the carbohydrate, little by little – watching both scales and clothes. You will find a level where you can eat as much as your body needs without gaining weight.

Appendix A
Dental Amalgam

Dental amalgam (sometimes called 'silver filling' in USA) is a mixture of 50% mercury to which has been added 35% silver and smaller amounts of tin, copper and zinc. Although its use has been written about as far back as the Middle Ages it didn't come into general use until the 19th century, and its present formulation is more or less unchanged since the beginning of the 20th century.

Because mercury is extraordinarily toxic – possibly the most poisonous of all non-radioactive metals – concerns have been raised from time to time by worried researchers. More recently, these still small voices have become more insistent and grown to become a great clamour. The increase in available knowledge, hitherto kept well out of public gaze by dental associations and dental manufacturers, has meant that the true facts are coming to light. In 1992 The International Academy of Oral Medicine and Toxicology (a professional organisation for dentists and dental research) wrote to all dental amalgam manufacturers saying, 'The potential for harmful health effects resulting from mercury exposure from mercury amalgam dental fillings is no longer a matter for scientific debate.'

The weak chemical bonding of the five metals used in dental amalgam means that the mercury may be leached out of the mixture as a result of pressure and heat, together with galvanic (electrical) interaction within the metallic mixture. The mercury vapour is taken up by the body, and it is estimated that an average amalgam filling releases about 10 micrograms of mercury daily. It turns out that two thirds of our mercury intake overall comes from this source. A further major derivation is from mercury waste. This is of great importance in dental clinics, where the waste may not be filtered and the mercury enters the food chain from sewage.

The big question therefore is not, does it happen, but what damage will it cause? Let us make a list.

1. Kidneys – the re-absorption mechanism is downgraded within the kidney tubules, reducing their efficiency. This in turn can lead to blood pressure and eventually renal failure.

2. There is an increased incidence of multiple intestinal antibiotic resistance. Effectively, therefore, the immune system becomes progressively compromised.

3. A large body of evidence has accumulated that mercury has a number of effects on the nervous system. It is now recognised that it acts as a neurotoxin, slowly weakening the nervous system. Mood, memory and motor function will be slowly degraded.

4. There are significant effects on fertility, which is reduced, but worse, it has been shown that there is a correlation existing with developmental abnormalities. Further work has demonstrated that mercury is passed to the baby in the womb, and after birth from breast milk.

5. A link has been found with cardiomyopathy, which is a progressive weakness of the muscles of the heart leading eventually to cardiac failure.

6. Studies on the role of trace elements in Alzheimer's disease have suggested that the raised levels of mercury could well be an important factor.

7. Thyroid and adrenal glands. Studies have shown that the thyroid/adrenal axis is down-regulated by mercury poisoning. The consequent symptomology will extend from mild to severe hypothyroidism and with adrenal involvement will have most if not all the features of the chronic fatigue syndrome. Many patients of my acquaintance have been much improved by the removal of their dental amalgam.

Dental practitioners and their associations and governing bodies have been largely dismissive of the dangers of mercury poisoning from dental amalgam. The vested interests of the dental manufacturers is a most powerful lobby, and has constantly stated that dental amalgam is perfectly safe, ignoring increasing evidence to the contrary. The almost unbelievable and disgraceful fact is that the American Dental Association takes disciplinary action, including loss of licence to practise, against dental practitioners who remove and replace dental amalgams. Other countries including the EU have campaigned constantly in favour of the use of dental amalgam, proclaiming that the evidence for its safety is irrefutable and cast iron. However, a wind of change is now gathering strength and Sweden, Norway, Germany, Denmark, Austria, Finland and Canada have recently taken steps to limit and phase out the use of amalgam fillings.

The removal of dental amalgam, and its replacement by ceramic fillings, however desirable, has to be done carefully and properly. The risk is inhalation and absorption of the mercury vapour in the removal process, and its being swallowed in the saliva. Most careful precautions have to be taken. If you propose to take this course of action, ensure that the dental surgeon has made a speciality of this work. Great care is needed to ensure that no accidental ingestion in any way occurs, and that waste amalgam is properly removed.

A word about the legal aspect. It was shown in 1992 that the American Dental Association (ADA) *'owes no legal duty of care to protect patients from the use of dental amalgam'*. The ADA has also made the removal of dental amalgam an 'issue of ethical conduct', and, as noted above, will proceed against dentists who recommend it. Further, the Food & Drug Administration (FDA) has *never* agreed on the use of mercury and silver *together*, i.e. as amalgam, although either may be used in combination with other metals.

The public outcry is such that the attitudes of these professional bodies are no longer acceptable, and if you suffer from chronic illness as we mentioned above, you may have yourself tested. There is a simple mouth test where a sensitive probe can pick up very small amounts of mercury vapour and a more complete test where the urine is measured after a challenge test of the dental amalgam. A chemical, DMPS, Dimaval, is given by mouth to release mercury from the system and measured in the urine before and after Dimaval is given. For more information I suggest that you check out www.amalgam.org, where you will find published references on which this Appendix is based. You should also see the excellent website of Dr Sukel – www.sukel.com.

If it becomes clear that you are indeed at risk you should present the evidence to your dentist or doctor and ask for referral to a specialist clinic.

Appendix B
Symptoms and Signs

Symptoms of Hypothyroidism

Constipation & flatulence

Depression

Anxiety

Poor sleep

Slow speech

Slow thinking

Memory loss

ADHD

Headaches

Thick tongue

Halitosis

Hoarse voice

Thickness of neck

Visual disturbances

Deafness & tinnitus

Ankle swelling

Puffy face & eyelids

Bladder irritation & frequency

Painful, irregular periods

Early menopause

Low fertility & loss of libido

Frequency of upper respiratory tract infections (URTI)

Frequency of urinary tract infections (UTI)

Fatigue - excessive tiredness

Muscle weakness

Weight gain

Shooting pains in hands and feet

Muscle & joint pain and stiffness

Breathlessness

Gallstones

Diminished sweating

Cold extremities

Intolerance to cold and heat

Pallor - yellowish tinge to skin

Bluish lips

Dry coarse skin

Brittle nails

Boils & spots

Eczema & psoriasis

Thinning hair

Loss of body hair

Loss of outer eyebrows

Candida

Haemorrhoids

Signs of Hypothyroidism

Loss of eyebrows	Hair loss
Skin problems	Cold hands and feet
Puffiness of eyes	Yellow skin
Low basal temperature	Slowed Achilles reflex
Soft and weakened pulse	Slow pulse
Goitre	Scalloped tongue
Umbilical hernia	Liver tenderness & enlargement
Albuminuria	Abdominal distension
Bruising	Clinical anaemia

The symptoms list is not exhaustive (although it is quite a good one), and you may well be able to add some for yourself. Some of the symptoms are also listed under signs, since these are things that are noticed by others – especially your doctor. One runs the risk, of course, of including every symptom and disability known to man, and thus go up one's own exhaust. As I said earlier, however, thyroid deficiency is the great pretender and any part of your system, in any combination with any other, may malfunction, producing its own particular mix of symptoms.

Symptoms of Low Adrenal Reserve

Weight loss	Poor response to thyroxine
Irritable bowel	Salt craving
Bowel upsets & diarrhoea	Sweet craving
Sensitivity to cold & heat	Hypoglycaemia
Cold extremities	Fainting attacks
Cold sweats	Poor response to infections
Dark rings under eyes	Repeated infections
Pigmentation in skin creases, gums	Breathlessness
Loss of body hair	Asthma

Generalised muscle weakness

Fatigue

Back & loin pain

Poor exercise tolerance

Palpitations

Aches & pains in muscles & joints

General depression and anxiety

Memory loss and confusion

Autoimmune disease

Hissing in ears

Internal shivering

Waking at night with:
  breathlessness, anxiety,
  sense of doom,
  hypoglycaemia

Signs of Low Adrenal Reserve

Prolonged or slow Achilles reflex

Raglan's sign (loss of blood
  pressure on standing)

Dark rings under eye

Loss of body hair

Breathlessness

Loss of hair on lower third of leg in men

Cold hands & feet

Dry thin skin

Skin pigmentation
  (of creases, gums, areolae)

Unstable pupillary reflex

Since low adrenal reserve is so often tied up with low thyroid states, you are likely to have a combination of both sets of symptoms; and as you can see, there is quite an overlap of symptoms anyway.

Appendix C
Assessment Charts

To help you make a decision and put into perspective a diagnosis of hypothyroidism and/or low adrenal reserve, I thought this chart might be helpful, not only for your personal use, but also in order to convince your doctor or any practitioner you consult.

Relevant Family Medical History

Mother...

....

....

Father...

....

....

Grandparents...

....

Aunts...

....

Uncles...

....

Cousins..

....

Personal Medical History

Past Illnesses...
....
....
Operations...
....
....
Major Life Events..
....

Summary of Present
Symptoms..
....
....
....
....
....
....
....
....
Signs..
....
....
....
....
....
....

Basal Temperature & Pulse Rates

Basal temperatures

Day 1	Day 2	Day 3	Day 4	Day 5	Day 6	Day 7
Day 8	Day 9	Day 10	Day 11	Day 12	Day 13	Day 14
Day 15	Day 16	Day 17	Day 18	Day 19	Day 20	Day 21
Day 22	Day 23	Day 24	Day 25	Day 26	Day 27	Day 28

Basal pulse rates

Day 1	Day 2	Day 3	Day 4	Day 5	Day 6	Day 7
Day 8	Day 9	Day 10	Day 11	Day 12	Day 13	Day 14
Day 15	Day 16	Day 17	Day 18	Day 19	Day 20	Day 21
Day 22	Day 23	Day 24	Day 25	Day 26	Day 27	Day 28

Appendix C

Test Results Chart

Test	Date/Result	Date/Result	Date/Result	Date/Result	Date/Result
FT4					
TT4					
FT3					
TT3					
TSH					
Thyroid Ab					
rT3					
FBC					
ESR					
LFT					
Ferritin					
Cholesterol					
Candida Ab					
DHEA					
Cortisol					
Adrenal Ab					
Oestrogen					
Progesterone					
Testosterone					

Appendix D
Resources, Useful Addresses & Further Reading

In the list below we have focused on UK organisations. Unfortunately we do not have the space to include this level of detail for the many other countries where we know this book will be read. However, if you have recommendations for additional links that should be added to the publisher's website please contact the publisher via www.hammersmithpress.co.uk.

Where to get your supplements

Glandulars & Nutritional Supplements
Nutri Ltd
Meridian House, Botany Business Park, Macclesfield Road, Whaley Bridge, High Peak, SK23 7DQ, UK.
Freephone Order Number: 0800 212 742   Freefax: 0800 371 731
email: orders@nutri.co.uk or info@nutri.co.uk

Glandulars & Nutritional Supplements
Nutri Centre
The Hale Clinic, 7 Park Crescent, London, W18 1PF, UK.
Tel: 00 44 (0)20 7436 5122   website: www.nutricentre.com

Armour Thyroid
Springfield Pharmacy
124 Sheen Road, Richmond, Surrey, TW9 1UL, UK.
Tel: 00 44 (0)20 8940 2304   Fax: 00 44 (0)20 8940 2661

Serenity Cream – Natural Progesterone
Triple Oestrogen Cream – Natural Oestrogen
Wellsprings Trading Ltd
PO Box 322, St Peter Port, Guernsey, GY1 3TP, Channel Islands.
Tel: 00 44 (0)1481 233 370   Fax: 00 44 (0)1481 235 206
website: www.progesterone.co.uk

Hormone Supplements
World Wide Health Corp
WWH Freepost, Alderney, GY1 5SS, Channel Islands.
Tel: 0800 952 9 952
website: www.wwhcorp.com email: customer_care@wwhcorp.com

Hormone Supplements
PharmWest
520 Washington Blvd #401, Marina del Rey, CA 90292, USA.
UK Freephone: 00800 8923 8923   Fax: 001 (310) 577 0296
website: www.pharmwest.com

Vitamins & Nutritional Support
Lamberts Healthcare Ltd
Lambert Road, Tunbridge Wells, Kent, TN2 3EH, UK.
Tel: 00 44 (0)1892 554312

Vitamins & Nutritional Support
Higher Nature
Burwash Common, East Sussex, TN19 7LX, UK.
Tel: 00 44 (0)1435 883702

Glandulars & Nutritional Supplements
Nutri-Meds Store
Nutri-Meds Inc, Corporate Office, 1704 Westland Road, Suite 8385,

Cheyenne, Wyoming 82001, USA.
website: www.nutri-meds.com   email: support@nutri-meds.com

Where to get tests done

All Tests
IWDL (Individual Wellbeing Diagnostic Laboratories)
Parkgate House, 356 West Barnes Lane, New Malden, Surrey, KT3 6NB, UK.
Tel: 00 44 (0)20 8336 7750   Fax: 00 44 (0)20 8336 7751   email: info@iwdl.net

All Tests
Red Apple Clinic (DiagnosTech) – Via Thyroid UK
32 Darcy Road, St Osyth, Clacton on Sea, Essex, CO16 8QF, UK.
website: www.thyroid.uk.org   email: enquiries@thyroiduk.org

Saliva & Blood
NPTech Services Ltd
Wellington House, Wellington Street, Newmarket, Suffolk, CB8 8SX, UK.
Tel: 00 44 (0)1638 665350   Fax: 01638 664913
website: www.NPTech.co.uk   email: info@NPTech.co.uk

Live Blood Analysis
Eagle Clinic – Dr Brian McDonogh (Live Blood Analysis, Holistic Medicine)
Milnwood House, 13 North Parade, Horsham, West Sussex, RH12 2BT, UK.
Tel: 00 44 (0)1403 258351   Fax: 00 44 (0)1403 258021
email: info@eagleclinic.com

Allergy Testing (Environmental Medicine & Nutrition)
The Burghwood Clinic – Dr John Mansfield
34 Brighton Road, Banstead, Surrey, SM7 1BS, UK.
Tel: 00 44 (0) 1737 361177   Fax: 00 44 (0) 1737 352245
Website: www.burghwoodclinic.co.uk   email: info@burghwoodclinic.co.uk

Reflexology
Tony Porter (LSCP. (phys) IIR (Regd) Hon) – Advanced Reflexology Training (ART)
28 Hollyfield Avenue, Friern Barnet, London, N11 3BY, UK.
Tel: 00 44 (0)208 368 0865   website: www.artreflex.com

Metabolic Diagnostic Advice & Nutritional Treatment
The Peatfield Clinic – Dr Barry Durrant-Peatfield
16 Southview Road, Warlingham, Surrey CR6 9JE, UK.
Tel/Fax: 00 44 (0)1883 623125   email: info@drpeatfield.com

Books for further reading

Hypothyroidism: The Unsuspected Illness – Broda O Barnes & Lawrence
Galton. (1976) Harper and Row ISBN: 0-690-01029
Available from The Barnes Foundation: www.brodabarnes.org

Solved: the Riddle of Illness – Stephen E Langer MD and James F Scheer.
(1995) Second Edition. Keats Publishing Inc ISBN 0-87983-667-9
Available from Amazon Books: www.amazon.com

Safe Uses of Cortisol – William McK Jefferies MD FACP.
(1996) Second Edition. Charles C Thomas ISBN 0-398-006621-3
Available from Amazon Books: www.amazon.com

From Fatigued to Fantastic – JacobTeitelbaum MD
(2001) Avery Publishing. ISBN 1-58333-097 6
Available from www.penguinputnam.com

The Metabolic Treatment of Fibromyalgia – Dr John C Lowe
(2000) McDowell Publishing. ISBN 0-914609-02-05
Available from: www.McDowellPublishing.com/ygmh.htm

Your Guide to Metabolic Health – Dr Gina Honeyman-Lowe & Dr John C Lowe
(2003) McDowell Publishing ISBN 0-974123-0-3
Available from: www.McDowellPublishing.com/ygmh.htm

Living Well With Hypothyroidism – Mary J Shomon
(2005) HarperCollins Publishers ISBN 0-0607-4095-7
Available from: www.thyroid.about.com

Living Well With Autoimmune Disease – Mary J Shomon
(2002) HarperCollins Publishers ISBN 0-0609-3819-6
Available from: www.autoimmunebook.com

Thyroid Power – Richard L Shames MD and Karilee Halo Shames
(2002) HarperCollins Publishers ISBN 0-688-17236-9
Available from Amazon Books: www.amazon.com

Dr Atkins New Diet Revolution – Robert C Atkins MD
(2002) Vermillion ISBN 0-09188-948-0
Available from his website: www.atkinscenter.com

The Miracle of Natural Hormones – David Brownstein MD
(1999) Second Edition. Medical Alternative Press
ISBN 0-9660882-0-4
Available from Amazon books: www.amazon.com

What Your Doctor May Not Tell You About Menopause – John R Lee MD
(2004) Little, Brown (USA) ISBN 0-446-67144-4
Available from Amazon books: www.amazon.com

Natural Progesterone – The Multiple Roles of a Remarkable Hormone
– John R Lee MD. (1999) BLL Publishing/Jon Carpenter, UK.
Available from Amazon books: www.amazon.com

Fluoride the Aging Factor – Dr John Yiamouyiannis
(1993) Third Edition. Health Action Press ISBN 0-913571-03-2
Available from NPWA: www.npwa.freeserve.co.uk

Fluoride: Drinking Ourselves to Death? – Barry Groves
(2001) New Leaf – Gill & Macmillan Ltd.
ISBN 0-7171-3274-9
Available from Amazon books: www.amazon.com

The Hormone Solution – Stay Younger Longer – Thierry Hertoghe MD
(2002) Random House. ISBN 0-609-60930-0
Available from Amazon books: www.amazon.com

Useful addresses & websites

Thyroid UK
32 Darcy Road, St Osyth, Clacton on Sea, Essex CO16 8QF, UK.
website: www.thyroid.uk.org   email: enquiries@thyroiduk.org

The Broda Barnes MD Research Foundation Inc
PO Box 98 Trumbull, Connecticut CT 06611, USA.
Tel: 001-203-261-2101 Fax: 001-102-261-3017
website: www.brodabarnes.org

Fibromyalgia Research Foundation
Dr John Lowe & Dr Gina Honeyman-Lowe
website: www.drlowe.com

Mary Shomon – Thyroid Support & Information
website: www.thyroid.about.com

Dr Rath – Fight Against Codex Alimentarius
website: www.dr-rath-foundation.org
email: vita-news@free-access-to-vitamins.net

Information About Amalgam
website: www.amalgam.org

Dr Sukel – Information About Amalgam
website: www.sukel.com

The Pituitary Foundation
PO Box 1944, Bristol BS99 2UB, UK.
Tel: 00 44 (0)1179 273355
website: www.pituitary.org.uk   email: helpline@pitpat.demon.co.uk

National Pure Water Association
website: www.npwa.freeserve.co.uk or www.fluoridealert.org

Thyroid Eye Disease Association (TED)
Solstice Sea Road, Winchelsea Beach, East Sussex TN36 4LH, UK.
Tel: 00 44 (0)1797 222338
website: www.thyroid-fed.org/members/TED.html

Thyroid Patient Advocacy – UK
PO Box 447, Keighley, BD22 OWR, UK.
website: www.tpa-uk.org.uk   email: info@tpa-uk.org.uk

Appendix E
References

Chapter Two

1. Lanni A, Moreno M, Lombardi A, Guglia F. Calorigenic effect of diiodothyronine in the rat. *Journal of Physiology* 1996; **494**: 831-837.

2. Horst C, Rokos H, Seitz HJ. Rapid stimulation of hepatic oxygen consumption by 3,5-di-iodo-L-thyronine. *Biochemical Journal.* 1989; **261**: 945-950.

3. Barnett CA, Visser TJ, Williams F, van Toor H, Duran S, Presas MJ, Morreale de Escobar, Hume R. Inadequate iodine intake of 40% of pregnant women from a region in Scotland. *Journal of Endocrinology Investigations* 2002; **25**(Suppl): 90.

Chapter Four

1. Flynn RWV, MacDonald TM, Morris AD. The Thyroid Epidemiology, Audit, and Research Study: Thyroid Dysfunction in the General Population. *Journal of Clinical Endocrinology & Metabolism* 2004; **89** (8) 3879-3884.

2. Masters R, Coplan M. Water Treatment with Silicofluorides and Lead Toxicity. *International Journal of Environmental Studies* 1999; **56**: 435-449.

3. Masters RD, Coplan MJ, Hone BT, Dykes JE. Association of Silicofluoride Treated Water with Elevated Blood Lead. *Neurotoxicology* 2000; **21**: 1101-1100.

4.   Coplan MJ, Masters RD, Hone B. Silicofluoride Usage, Tooth Decay and Children's Blood Lead. Poster presentation to *Conference on Environmental Influences on Children: Brain, Development and Behavior*, New York Academy of Medicine, Mt. Sinai Hospital, New York, 1999; May 24-25.

5.   Goldman GS, Yazbak FE. An investigation of the association between MMR vaccination and autism in Denmark. *Journal of American Physicians and Surgeons* 2002; **9** (3): 70-75.

6.   Li SX, Zh JL, Gao RD. Effect of high fluoride water supply on children's intelligence. *Fluoride* 1996; **29** (4): 190-192.

7.   Mullenix PJ, Denbesten PK, Schunior A, Kernan WJ. Neurotoxicity of Sodium Fluoride in Rats. *Journal of Neurotoxicology and Teratology* 1995; 17:169-177.

8.   Mullenix PJ. *CNS damage from fluorides*. (14th Sept 1998) http://www.cadvision.com/fluoride/brain2.htm

9.   Editorial. Chronic Fluoride Intoxication. *JAMA* Sept 18 1943; **123**:150.

10. Aardema, Marilyn J et al. Sodium Fluoride -induced Chromosome Aberrations in Different Stages of the Cell Cycle: A Proposed Mechanism. *Mutation Research* 1989; **223**:191-203.

11. He H, Chen ZS, Liu XM. The effects of fluoride on the human embryo. *Chinese Journal of Control of Epidemic Diseases* 1989; **4**: 136-137.

12. Spittle B, Ferguson D, Bouwer C. Intelligence and fluoride exposure in New Zealand children. Abstracts of papers to be presented at the *XXIInd Conference of the International Society for Fluoride Research* August 1998; S13: 24-27.

13. Hashimoto H. Zur kenntnis der lymphomatosen veranderung der schilddruse (struma lymphomatosol). *Archiv der Klinische Chirurgie* 1912; **97** :21.

14.   Kuhr T, Hala K, Dietrich H, Herold M, Wick G. Genetically determined target organ susceptibility in the pathogenesis of spontaneous autoimmune thyroiditis: aberrant expression of MHC-class II antigens and the possible role of virus. *Journal of Autoimmunity* 1994; **7** :13-25.

15.   Durrant-Peatfield BJ. Aspects of a Common Missed Diagnosis: Thyroid Dysfunction and Management. *Journal of Nutritional & Environmental Medicine* 1996; **6** (4): 371-378.

16.   Leckie RG, Buckner AB, Borneman, M. Seatbelt related thyroiditis documented with thyroid Te-99m perlechnetate scans. *Clinical Nuclear Medicine* 1992; **17** (11): 859-660.

17.   Lowe JC. *The Metabolic Treatment of Fibromyalgia*. USA: McDowell Publishing; 2000.

Chapter Five

1.   Weiner H. Emotions and Mentation. In: *The Thyroid*. Fourth Edition. USA: Harper & Row; 1987.

2.   Gewirtz GR, Malaspina D, Hattener JA, Feureisen S, Klein D, Gorman JM. Occult thyroid dysfunction in patients with refractory depression. *American Journal of Psychiatry* 1998; **145** (8): 1012-1014.

3.   Schatz IJ, Masaki K, Yano K *et al.* Cholesterol and all-cause mortality in elderly people from the Honolulu Heart Program: A cohort study. *Lancet* 2001; **358**: 351-355.

4.   Turner KB, Present CH, Bidwell EH. The thyroid in the regulation of the blood cholesterol in rabbits. *Journal Experimental Medicine*. 1938; **67**: 111.

5.   Barnes BO, Galton L. *Hypothyroidism: The Unsuspected Illness*. USA: Harper and Row; 1976.

6.   Derry D. *Breast Cancer and Iodine: How to Prevent and How to Survive Breast Cancer*. Canada: Trafford Publishing; 2001.

Chapter Six

1. Schnert KW, Croft AC. Basal Metabolic temperature versus laboratory assessment in post traumatic hypothyroidism. *Journal of Manipulative and Physiological Therapeutics* 1996; **19** (1): 6-12.

2. Wartofsky L, Dickey R. Perspective: The Evidence for a Lower Reference Range for Thyrotropin (TSH) is Compelling. 2006. *The American Association of Clinical Endocrinologists.* www.aace.com.

3. Heydarian P, Azizi F. The frequency of thyroid antibodies is higher in the upper range of normal thyrotropin values. *International Journal of Endocrinology and Metabolism* 2005; **1**: 10-17.

4. Baisier WV, Hertoghe T, Eeckhaut. Thyroid Insufficiency. Is TSH measurement the only diagnostic tool? *Journal of Environmental Medicine* 2000; **10**: 105.

5. Furmaniak J, Smith BR. Immunity to the Thyroid Stimulating Hormone Receptor. *Springer Seminars in Immunopathology* 1993; **14**: 309-321.

Chapter Seven

1. Barnes BO, Galton L. *Hypothyroidism: The Unsuspected Illness.* First Edition. USA: Harper and Row; 1976.

2. Venturi S. Is there a role for iodine in breast diseases? *The Breast* 2001; **10** (5): 379-382.

3. Ghent WR, Eskin BA, Low DA, Hill LP. Iodine replacement in fibrocystic disease of the breast. *Canadian Journal of Surgery* 1993; **36**: 453-460

4. Derry D. *Breast Cancer and Iodine: How to Prevent and How to Survive Breast Cancer.* Canada: Trafford Publishing; 2001.

5. Eskin BA. Dietary iodine and cancer risk. *Lancet.* 1976; **8**: 807-808.

6.   Singh BB, Simpson RL. Incidence of Premenstrual Syndrome and Remedy Usage: A National Probability Sample Study. *Alternative Therapies in Health and Medicine* 1998; **3**: 75-79.

7.   Majeed A, Babb P, Jones J, Quinn M. Trends in prostate cancer incidence, mortality and survival in England and Wales 1971-1998. *British Journal of Urology International* 2000; **85** (9): 1058-1062.

8.   Rupprecht R. The neuropsychopharmacological potential of neuroactive steroids. *Journal of Psychiatric Research* 1997; **31** (3): 297-314.

9.   Stemberg TH, le Van P, Wright ET. The hydrating effects of pregnenolone acetate on the human skin. *Current Therapeutic Research* 1961; **3** (11): 469-471.

10.   Schwartz A. DHEA extends lifespan. Presentation at The New York Academy of Science Conference on DHEA. June 1995.

11.   Schwartz AG, Pashko LL. Dehydroepiandrosterone, glucose-6-phosphate dehydrogenase, and longevity. *Ageing Research Reviews* 2004; **3** (2): 171-187.

12.   Helzlsouer KJ, Gordon GB, Alberg AH et al. Relationship of prediagnostic serum levels of dehydroepiandrosterone and dehydroepiandrosterone sulfate to the risk of developing premenopausal breast cancer. *Cancer Research* 1992; **52**: 1-4.

13.   Barrett-Connor E, Friedlander NJ, Khaw KT. Dehydroepiandrosterone sulfate and breast cancer risk. *Cancer Research* 1990; **50** (20): 6571-6574.

14.   Morales A et al. Effects of replacement dose of DHEA in men and women of advancing age. *Journal of Clinical Endocrinology & Metabolism* 1994; 78: 1360-1367.

15.   Rasmussen KR, Henley MC, Cheng L, Yang S. Effects of dehydroepiandrosterone in immunosuppressed adult mice infected with cryptosporidium parvum. *Journal of Parasitology* 1995; 81(3): 429-433.

16.   Hertoghe T. *The Hormone Solution*. USA: Harmony Books; 2002: 160-161.

17.   Pierpaoli W, Regelsen W. Pineal control of ageing: effect of melatonin and pineal grafting on ageing mice. *Proceedings of the National Academy of Science, USA* 1994; **94**: 787-791.

18.   Reiter RJ et al. Melatonin and its relation to the immune system and inflammation. *Annals of the New York Academy of Science* 2000; **917**: 376-386.

19.   Reiter RJ. Historical Account of the Research Related to EMF, Melatonin and Cancer. Presentation at *Symposium 2000: Low frequency EMF, Visible Light, Melatonin and Cancer*.

20.   Papayasiliou PS, Duby SE, Steck AJ, Bell M, Lawrence, WH. Melatonin and Parkinsonism. *JAMA* 1972; **221** (1): 88.

Chapter Nine

1.   Flynn RWV, MacDonald TM, Morris AD. The Thyroid Epidemiology, Audit, and Research Study: Thyroid Dysfunction in the General Population. *Journal of Clinical Endocrinology & Metabolism* 2004; **89** (8): 3879-3884.

2.   Barnes BO, Galton L. *Hypothyroidism: The Unsuspected Illness*. USA, Harper and Row; 1976.

3.   American Association of Clinical Endocrinologists. *Thyroid Undercover hiding in plain sight*. Thyroid Awareness Month 2003 www.aace.com/public/awareness/tam/2003

4.   Pauling L. *Vitamin C, the Common Cold, and the Flu*. USA, W H Freeman & Co. 1976.

5.   Honeyman-Lowe G. Vitamin C - How much and how often? *Metabolic Health Newsletter*. 1997; (Nov 5): 1-3.

6. Shomon M. (2006 update) *More Levoxyl Recalls - July 2002. Almost 3 Million Levoxyl Tablets Recalled.* www.thyroid-info.com/articles/ levoxyl12.htm

Chapter Fourteen

1. Eaton CD. Co-existence of hypothyroidism with diabetes mellitus. *Journal of Michigan Medical Society* 1954; **53**: 1101.

Chapter Fifteen

1. Friedland IB. Investigations on the Influence of Thyroid Preparations on Experimental Hypercholesterolemia and Atherosclerosis. *Zeitung Ges Exp Med* 1933; **87**: 683.

2. Turner KB et al. The role of the thyroid in the regulation of the blood cholesterol of rabbits. *Journal of Experimental Medicine* 1938; **67**: 111.

3. Barnes BO, Barnes CW. *Heart Attack Rareness in Thyroid-Treated Patients.* USA, Charles C Thomas Publisher; 1972: 75.

4. Brody J. Statins: Miracles for some, menace for a few. *New York Times* Personal Health Column. December 2002.

5. Chazerain P, Hayem G, Hamza S, Best C, Ziza JM. Four Cases of Tendinopathy in Patients on Statin Therapy. *Joint Bone Spine* 2001; **68** (5): 430-433.

6. Evans M, Rees A. The myotoxicity of statins. *Current Opinion in Lipidology* 2002; **13** (4): 415-420.

7. Hodel C. Myopathy and rhabdomyolysis with lipid-lowering drugs. *Toxicology Letters* 2002; **128**(1-3): 159-168.

8. Bodansky M, Bodansky O. *The Biochemistry of Diseases.* USA, The Macmillan Company; 1940: 341.

Chapter Sixteen

1. Joffe RT. A perspective of the thyroid and depression. *Canadian Journal of Psychiatry* 1990; **35**: 374-378.

2. Hebert LE, Scherr PA, Bienias JL, Bennett DA, Evans DA. Alzheimer Disease in the US Population: Prevalence Estimates Using the 2000 Census. *Archives of Neurology* 2003; **60**(8): 1119-1112.

Chapter Seventeen

1. Rudman D, Feller AG, Nagraj HS, Gergans GA, Lalitha PY, Goldberg AF, Schlenker RA, Cohn L, Rudman IW, Mattson DE. Effects of human growth hormone in men over 60 years old. *New England Journal of Medicine* 1990; **323**(1):1-6.

Chapter Eighteen

1. Baisier WV, Hertoghe T, Eeckhaut W. Thyroid Insufficiency. Is TSH measurement the only diagnostic tool? *Journal of Environmental Medicine* 2000; **10**: 105.

Chapter Nineteen

1. Demers LM, Spencer CA. Laboratory Support for the Diagnosis and Monitoring of Thyroid Disease. *Thyroid* 2003; **13**: 57-58.

2. Fatourechi V, Klee GG, Grebe SK et al. Effects of reducing the upper limit of normal TSH values. *JAMA* 2003; **290**: 3195-3196.

3. Heydarian P, Azizi F. The Frequency of Thyroid Autoantibodies is Higher in the Upper Range of Normal Thyrotropin Values. *International Journal of Endocrinology & Metabolism* 2005; **1**: 10-17.

4. Stephens PA. Current Issues in Thyroid Disease Management. *Endocrine News* 2004; **2** 9:2.

Appendix E

General References

Atkins RC. *Dr Atkins New Diet Revolution*. UK: Vermillion; 2002.

Barnes BO, Galton L. *Hypothyroidism: The Unsuspected Illness*. USA: Harper and Row; 1976.

Brownstein D. *The Miracle of Natural Hormones*. Second Edition. USA: Medical Alternative Press; 1999.

Groves B. *Fluoride: Drinking Ourselves to Death?* Dublin: New Leaf - Gill & Macmillan Ltd; 2001.

Hertoghe T. *The Hormone Solution*. USA: Random House; 2002.

Holford P. *The H Factor*. UK: Judy Piatkus (Publishers) Ltd; 2003.

Holford P. *Optimum Nutrition for the Mind*. UK: Judy Piatkus (Publishers) Ltd; 2003.

Holford P. *The Holford Low GL Diet*. UK: Judy Piatkus (Publishers) Ltd; 2005.

Langer SE, Scheer JF. *Solved the Riddle of Illness*. Second Edition. USA: Keats Publishing Inc; 1995.

Lee JR. *Natural Progesterone: The Multiple Roles of a Remarkable Hormone*. USA: BLL Publishing; 1999.

Lowe JC. *Metabolic Treatment of Fibromyalgia*. USA: McDowell Publishing; 2000.

McK Jefferies W. *Safe Uses of Cortisol*. Second Edition. Charles C Thomas; 1996.

Puri BK. *Chronic Fatigue Syndrome - a natural way to treat M.E.* London: Hammersmith Press; 2005.

Teitelbaum J. *From Fatigued to Fantastic*. Avery Publishing.

Yiamouyiannis J. *Fluoride the Aging Factor*. Third Edition. USA: Health Action Press; 1993.

Index

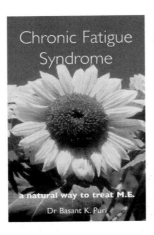

Chronic Fatigue Syndrome - a way to treat M.E.
By Professor Basant K Puri
160pp   £14.99
ISBN: 1-905140-00-2
Publication: January 2005 (Revised reprint January 2006)

Whoever the ME sufferer, young or old, man or woman, he or she is likely to have been told the condition is 'psychosomatic' or 'all in the mind', depression is the root cause, and antidepressants the only sensible answer.

In this ground-breaking new book you will discover a very different way of looking at M.E. Professor Puri brings together historical and contemporary evidence to show how M.E. is almost certainly a physical, or 'organic' condition resulting from viral and other influences that reduce essential chemicals in the body. As such, it can be treated, and in a natural cost effective way.

Read how and why EPA ('eicosapentaenoic acid') will be essential to recovery, how to take it, what supplements to have with it, and how to change to a lifestyle that will promote recovery.

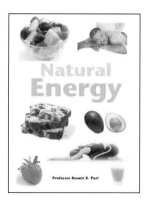

Natural Energy
By Professor Basant K Puri
224 pp   £12.99
ISBN: 1-905140-02-9
Due for publication: October 2009

Extending the principles of treating M.E. and ADHD with a diet rich in phospholipids to the promotion of greater energy in any individual. Modern lifestyles are blamed for increasing tiredness experienced by the general population but poor diet has a significant role to play and there are clear ways to combat this trend and increase personal levels of physical and mental energy. Professor Puri explains what factors inhibit our bodies' healthy use of essential fatty acids and what factors do the reverse and why our ability to process omega-3 and omega-6 fatty acids effectively has such a profound effect on our health.

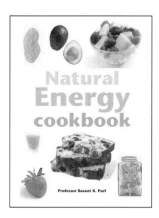

The Natural Energy Cookbook
By Professor Basant Puri
Cookery advisor: Sarah Banbery
224 pp   £14.99
ISBN: 1-905140-03-7
Due for publication: October 2009

The practical way to achieve a diet high in phospho-lipids that is also delicious, varied and easy to prepare. Grouped around key ingredients, the book presents tried-and-tested recipes together with weekly menu plans. This is the 'how to do it' counterpart of 'Natural Energy', putting theory into practice in an attractively clear, and delicious, way.

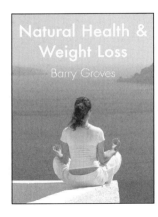

Natural Health & Weight Loss
By Barry Groves
224 pp £12.99
ISBN: 1-905140-15-0
Publication: April 2007

Recognizing that the epidemic of obesity in the western world has coincided with 'Health Eating' recommendations, Barry Groves brings together a huge body of research, and experience, to show what we are doing wrong. He sets out how we have to overcome our now ingrained prejudices against fat in favour of whole-grains and fruit in order to regain our long term health and natural body weight.